Explorations in Psychiatric Sociology

Edited by

PAUL M. ROMAN

Associate Professor, Department of Sociology
Newcomb College, Tulane University
New Orleans, Louisiana

HARRISON M. TRICE

Professor, Department of Organizational Behavior
New York State School of Industrial and Labor Relations
Cornell University
Ithaca, New York

F. A. DAVIS COMPANY, PHILADELPHIA

Library of Congress Cataloging in Publication Data

Roman, Paul M.
  Explorations in psychiatric sociology.

  Includes bibliographies.
  1. Social psychiatry. I. Trice, Harrison Miller, 1920-   joint author. II. Title. [DNLM: 1. Psychiatry, Community. WM440 R758e 1974]
  BF455.R578   616.8'9'071   74-8345
  ISBN 0-8036-7550-X

To
Professor Alfred McClung Lee

Exemplar of the founding
spirit of the Society for
the Study of Social Problems

Preface

The interrelations between mental illness and the social milieu have long been of interest to sociologists. The repeated implications that aberrant behavior and communication have roots in socialization processes have attracted much research effort. The existing range of institutional forms dealing with mental illness has been a subject of sociological analysis. Indeed, the past decade has seen the emergence of a quasi-social movement which has challenged psychiatric theory and practice, bringing into focus social and cultural constructions in what are officially regarded as psychological species of human disease.

The development of a distinctive subspecialty of psychiatric sociology has been a rather slow and fitful process, despite the scope of sociological interest in the genesis and control of mental illness. Included in this volume are a range of perspectives from specialists in psychiatric sociology which outline the theoretical and methodological approaches in the sociological study of psychiatric phenomena and illustrate the application of these approaches to four substantive categories of psychiatric problems. The book is not intended to provide comprehensive coverage of the issues and data generated by psychiatric sociologists, but rather to sensitize both the scholar and the student to the excitement as well as the dilemmas that characterize this area of scientific endeavor.

This book and its companion, *Sociological Perspectives in Community Mental Health* (Philadelphia: F.A. Davis, 1974), are official projects of the Society for the Study of Social Problems, an organization of sociologists formed in the early 1950's to focus sociological expertise on the real world issues of modern society. The project began when the editors were co-chairpersons on the Society's Division of Psychiatric Sociology, when Division members agreed that these volumes would provide a useful contribution consistent with the Society's objectives. To a degree, this volume represents an up-dating of a 1955 volume sponsored by the S.S.S.P. and edited by Arnold Rose, *Mental Health and Mental Disorder*. All royalties from the sale of these books will go to the Society to support its activities.

The chapters are original to this book. We are grateful to the contributors for making this project a rewarding experience for us, and their generosity in contributing their efforts for the benefit of the S.S.S.P. is deeply appreciated.

We are indebted to Hyman Rodman, past chairperson of the S.S.S.P. Editorial and Publication Committee, who took many hours during a sabbatical leave to assure publication of the volume, and to Joe D. Witcher and Irma Agnew of the F. A. Davis Company for their considerable help in arranging the details of publication. Christine Young did a superior job of editing and improving the manuscript, and her patience in dealing with the editors is most appreciated. Finally, as editors, colleagues, and co-participants in a very durable friendship, we express gratitude to each other for endurance, optimism, and occasional flashes of sound judgement that helped make this effort a reality.

P.M.R.
H.M.T.

Contributors

PAULINE B. BART, Abraham Lincoln Medical School, University of Illinois, Chicago, Illinois

JAMES D. CAMPBELL, Coe College, Cedar Rapids, Indiana

C. R. FLETCHER, Eastern Virginia Medical School, Norfolk, Virginia

ROBERT M. GRAY, University of Utah, Salt Lake City, Utah

JAMES M. HENSLIN, Southern Illinois University, Edwardsville, Illinois

MELVIN L. KOHN, Laboratory of Socioenvironmental Studies, National Institute of Mental Health, Bethesda, Maryland

PETER K. MANNING, Michigan State University, East Lansing, Michigan

MICHAEL MOORE, University of California, Davis, California

ADINA M. REINHARDT, Salt Lake City Community Mental Health Center, Salt Lake City, Utah

LARRY T. REYNOLDS, Central Michigan University, Mount Pleasant, Michigan

LEE N. ROBINS, Washington University, St. Louis, Missouri

CONSTANTINA SAFILIOS-ROTHSCHILD, Wayne State University, Detroit, Michigan

JAMES O. SMITH, University of Wisconsin, Milwaukee, Wisconsin

LEO SROLE, Columbia University, New York, New York

S. KIRSON WEINBERG, Loyola University, Chicago, Illinois

Contents

Part I - Definition of the Field 2

Chapter 1
Sociology and Psychiatry: Fusions and Fissions of Identity 5
    Leo Srole

Part II - Theory and Method in Psychiatric Sociology

Introduction 20

Chapter 2
Issues in the Scope and Theory of Psychiatric Sociology 25
    S. Kirson Weinberg

Chapter 3
The Labeling Theory and Mental Illness 43
    C. R. Fletcher, Peter K. Manning, Larry T. Reynolds,
    and James O. Smith

Chapter 4
The Search for the Causes of Psychiatric Disorder 63
    Lee N. Robins

Chapter 5
Problems of Cross-Cultural Research in Psychiatric Sociology 81
    Constantina Safilios-Rothschild, and Michael Moore

Part III - Research in Psychiatric Sociology

Introduction 106

Chapter 6
Social Class and Schizophrenia: A Critical
    Review and a Reformulation 113
      Melvin L. Kohn

Chapter 7
The Sociology of Depression 139
      Pauline B. Bart

Chapter 8
Sociology and the Study of Suicide 159
      James M. Henslin, and James D. Campbell

Chapter 9
Adjustment to Society: Interrelations Among
    Anomia, Social Class, and Psychiatric Impairment 185
      Adina M. Reinhardt, and Robert M. Gray

Index 209

Part I

DEFINITION OF THE FIELD

Psychiatric sociology represents a sociological specialty that has been rapidly burgeoning. Aside from other testimony, the level of activity and interest in the Division on Psychiatric Sociology of the Society for the Study of Social Problems is evidence of this trend. While the bases for this growth have not been studied by sociologists of science, several factors appear to account for the emergence of interest in this specialty.

The problem of mental illness remains significant to both policymakers and the public. Mass media efforts have probably increased the public's awareness and concern about mental illness in the past decade. Whether the incidence of mental illness is increasing remains debatable, although such a hypothesis is attractive with jeremiads on all sides bewailing the troubles of the times. To some, these troubles are causes of increased emotional disorder, while to others, the prevalence of emotional disorder in the population is viewed as leading to varying degrees of social disintegration. While problems in the establishment of causality, as well as means of measuring true prevalence, are dealt with in this book, it is sufficient to say that mental illness is a significant public issue, a fact which has set the stage for the emergence of psychiatric sociology.

Stemming from this public prominence and the pragmatic orientation to action which characterizes American social policy, it is logical to expect that attacks on the problem will be supported on many fronts. Sociologists have increasingly participated in the search for the causes of mental illness, studying the operation of health care delivery systems for psychiatric disorders with the goal of enhancing their effectiveness, and offering their students the research skills and substantive knowledge necessary for furthering basic and applied research in this area. The nature of this support has changed over time with different policy emphases at the federal level, but available financial support must be a central explanation for the emergence and growth of psychiatric sociology.

Available financial support is, however, far from a total explanation of the sociological interest in mental disorders. Behavioral scientists find the phenomenon of mental illness fascinating and in need of explanation. With normal behavior seemingly characterizing most people, why is it that some individuals withdraw, or are withdrawn, from social participation through modes of behavior which often defy the imagination by their content and unpredictability? The delineation of predisposing factors and their respective linkages is a challenge to the theories of human behavior; moreover, it is frequently stated that an understanding of abnormal behavior may lead us closer to a more complete theory of normal behavior.

The methodological challenges involved in studying mental illness are many. Much research has been reported at the clinical level, leading the sociologist to question the representative nature of the data on which numerous hypotheses have been based. To many sociologists, the study of mental disorder calls for appropriate types of survey research to assure representativeness, and at the same time calls for data collection techniques which must be aimed not only at defining a case of mental illness, but also at the collection of background and current data which are both valid and reliable. Together, these theoretical and methodological challenges are bound to broaden issues in sociology, making the study of psychiatric disorders potentially fruitful for the building of social theory and the refinement of methodological techniques.

Aside from the guidance to "significant" research questions provided by the patterning of available research funds, the field of sociology has been recently marked by challenges to its relevance. Furthermore, there has been sharp concern about controlling the social impact of research procedures and results. Some sociologists have accused their colleagues of consorting with the power structure and conducting research with implications that are either supportive of the status quo, or benign and inane. While the 20 plus years of vigorous existence of the Society for the Study of Social Problems challenges the novelty of relevant research concerns, this issue has sharpened in recent years. The concern over relevance has made psychiatric sociology an attractive specialty with some tendencies to overplay the "underdog" status of psychiatric patients.

The social institution of psychiatry and its modes of operation have provided many points for attack by sociologists. Here the concern with relevance has been manifest in studies of the labeling process involved in psychiatric diagnosis and treatment, and its subsequent role in the creation of chronic mental illness. These studies have set the stage for a lively debate in sociology regarding the validity of the research implications generated by the labeling theorists' results.

In this book, we attempt to highlight these developments through the use of five essays dealing with theory and methodology, followed by summaries of research in four substantive areas. This collection is not intended to be exhaustive, but rather it constitutes a sampling of issues which collectively provide a profile of the current status of psychiatric sociology.

The term *psychiatric sociology* creates considerable confusion about the specialty's scope and emphasis. It is often confused with the terms *social psychiatry, psychiatric social work* or with *therapeutic sociology,* i.e., direct efforts by sociologists to enhance the mental health status of a population through the application of behavioral science theory. While somewhat cumbersome, the designation appears to be the best one developed to date. Other terms such as *the sociology of psychiatry,* or *the sociology of mental disorders,* or *the sociology of mental health* are rejected because of their narrow scope since the field encompasses research and theory on both discrete mental disorders and the various modes of psychiatric practice.

More profound confusion emerges when psychiatric sociology is compared with social psychiatry. The latter term applies to a diffuse psychiatric specialty concerned primarily with intervention, but also involved in research activities which overlap and even duplicate those carried out by sociologists. It is appropriate that our first chapter is focused upon this issue. It is also appropriate that the author is Leo Srole, a pioneer psychiatric sociologist, who has conducted numerous research efforts involved with such issues as case definition, etiology, and intervention. Srole is further qualified by the fact that most of his career activities

3

have been carried out within medical settings. His ability to sustain a bridging function is marked by his being the only sociologist ever elected an Honorary Fellow of the American Psychiatric Association.

In his chapter, Srole undertakes to clarify the boundaries and areas of overlap between social psychiatry and psychiatric sociology. Srole's chapter represents a unique effort to logically derive the content of psychiatric sociology. The term social psychiatry is often used to encapsulate the concerns of psychiatric sociology, implying that this use of sociological theory and methods is rightfully the province of psychiatry by virtue of psychiatry's mandate over the entire field of psychiatric disorder. As a sociologist, Srole does not defensively carve out sociology's specific jurisdiction. Rather he focuses upon the competencies of the two fields as a basis for appropriate scopes of work.

Many contemporary sociologists would take issue with Srole's encouragement that sociologists work side by side with the psychiatrist. As mentioned, many sociologists whose work is focused upon mental illness, particularly those employing the labeling perspective, view psychiatry as an insidious system of social control and want no part of efforts designed to improve the effectiveness of psychiatry's operations. It is also obvious that interdisciplinary activities of the type Srole proposes contain the potential for interprofessional conflict. Whether the psychiatrist is willing to recognize the sociologist as a professional with standing equal to his own, and as a professional with a unique set of skills, has been shown to be problematic. Nearly all interdisciplinary efforts take place within a setting dominated by psychiatrists rather than by sociologists, e.g., one is hard pressed to find psychiatrists among the staff members of sociology departments, whereas numerous sociologists are employed by academic departments of psychiatry. Thus, the sociologist who attempts to carry out a role on an interdisciplinary team dominated by psychiatrists frequently finds his efforts sharply controlled and his status sometimes reduced to that of a minion.

Despite these problems in Srole's prescriptions, his chapter comprises a position paper which is based in the real world. His emphasis upon professional competence as being the basis for determining the division of labor is indeed worthy of greater attention. Both sociologists and psychiatrists are guilty of carelessly using each other's concepts and methods without adequate consideration of who is best equipped to carry out certain research tasks.

CHAPTER 1

Sociology and Psychiatry: Fusions and Fissions of Identity*

LEO SROLE†

The Theodorsons' *Modern Dictionary of Sociology* identifies a long list of subspecialties within sociology, but does not include psychiatric sociology among them. Its absence is not altogether surprising. This subspecialty had its first conceptual stirrings in the years before World War I and its launch as a substantive field of research in the threshold years of World War II.[5] Until recently, however, sociologists who ventured into this opening frontier were content in the main to align themselves with psychiatrists in staking out this borderland under the designation of *social psychiatry*.

As signs of its institutional stature, social psychiatry has since had its name taken into the titles of world congresses, international journals, numerous monographs, and innumerable professional symposia. Yet we are confronted with the striking anomaly that beneath these impressive organizational trappings, elementary controversies continue to boil as to what substantive content is in fact, or should by definition be in the semantic vessel called social psychiatry.

I cite three instances of this definitional ambiguity. Morris Carstairs, a prominent psychiatrist, declared on a recent professional occasion: "All I know is that what I mean by social psychiatry, and what Maxwell Jones, or Moreno, or even Gerald Caplan mean by the same words, amount to very different concepts." On that occasion psychiatrist Fritz Freyhan stated more pointedly:

---

*Adapted from "Social Psychiatry: A Case of the Babel Syndrome", an invited paper read to the American Psychopathological Association annual meetings of 1967 and published in Zubin and Freyhan.[15]

†The author's current research is being carried out in the Columbia University Psychiatry Department's Social Sciences Research Unit. His work has been supported since 1967 by a grant from the National Institute of Mental Health to the unit's program in psychiatric sociology. The program's purpose is to clarify and advance the potentialities of this young sociological research field.

5

"Social psychiatry has become everybody's excuse for thinking or doing as one pleases." A third instance is provided by John Clausen, a sociologist. One of the editors of a wide-ranging book, published in 1957, entitled *Explorations in Social Psychiatry,* his current view was expressed on the same recent occasion: "Social psychiatry is, for this sociologist, an extremely ambiguous and unsatisfactory concept for delineating a field of scholarly investigation."

I too have had publications which I identified as falling within the domain of social psychiatry. Subsequently, I joined others who were becoming concerned about the field's increasing state of disarray, which I then interpreted as being largely rooted in the diversity of its theoretical origins. Several years ago, however, I came to the conclusion that this etiological view was rather less than the whole story. In a new interdisciplinary field, conceptual diversities are desirable and, in fact, inevitable. But if in the course of considerable time, there is a progressive falling out instead of some consolidation of conceptual ranks, then it seems likely that some other kind of aggravating factor is intruding. It becomes clear to me that perhaps we had not come to grips with our original conceptual differences, in part because they were obscured by cross-cutting difficulties on the more superficial level of contending labels—i.e., of competing nomenclatures.

I was subsequently pleased to find a kindred view held by Bell and Spiegel.[2] Their paper is illuminating in uncovering the somewhat separate roller-coaster histories of the term social psychiatry within American psychiatry and sociology since 1917. They also draw what is surely one of the most qualified conclusions in the entire scientific literature: "The coherence (if there is any) of this field (if it is one) is notably difficult to discover."

However had they carried their analysis one step farther, they would have discovered that the incoherence discerned is not without some structure. From their own data and Goldston's[6] selected definitions, it becomes evident that over its 50-year history, social psychiatry has been a label fluidly applied within the space of two major, cross-cutting semantic dimensions, as represented in Figure 1.

The X axis refers to the discipline(s) identified with social psychiatry. The Y

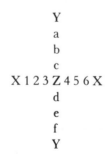

Figure 1
The Dimensions of "Social Psychiatry."

axis refers to function(s) identified with social psychiatry. Z is the unoccupied intersection point of the two axes.

Each dimension in Figure 1 is schematically and arbitrarily arranged as if there were six identifiable points of semantic variation on its entire range of historical differences. Most users of the term since 1917 can be variously located at points on both dimensions simultaneously. However, in the interest of brevity and clarity I shall have to discuss the two axes separately.

The X axis represents the *disciplines* identifed with social psychiatry. For example, Point 1 might denote those clinicians who have contended that social psychiatry, however functionally defined, is exclusively a domain of and for psychiatrists. Point 2 could refer to those who have seen social psychiatry embodied in the working team of the clinician and psychiatric social worker as senior and junior members respectively. Point 3 would be held for those classifying social psychiatry as a subspecialty of psychiatry in which social scientists have a place, albeit in a more or less ancillary technical role. Point 4 is reserved for those defining social psychiatry as a joint enterprise of psychiatrists and social scientists as equal partners. Point 5 then denotes those who differentiate social psychiatry as of joint *substantive* interest to the two older disciplines, but at least methodologically belonging in the field of the social sciences. Finally, around Point 6 might be gathered the early generation of sociologists who claimed social psychiatry as exclusively a social science preserve. This view persists in a slightly altered form among advocates of the ostensibly new subspecialty called *clinical sociology.*

The Y axis refers to variations in the *service versus research* functions identified with social psychiatry. For example, the upper half of the range (a, b, c) embraces all those who assign only the service function to social psychiatry, but who vary in the nature and magnitude of the services to be performed. For example, at point "a" stand those who classify a social psychiatrist in the minimal terms of the one-to-one relationship therapist who, in diagnosis and treatment, systematically takes into account sociocultural aspects of the patient's life setting. At point "c" are those who see the social psychiatrist as a therapist primarily to groups or societies as entities rather than to individual patients. At intervening point "b" would fall those who equate social psychiatry with manipulation of groups in the service of the patient—for example, milieu therapy, the therapeutic community, and family treatment.

On the other half of the Y axis, social psychiatry is largely identified with the research function. For example, point "d" might refer to therapy-process studies of a one-to-one dyad, and point "f" to basic etiological investigations of large, general populations. Explorations of psychiatric treatment institutions, or of patient families would cluster around intervening point "e".

To specifically illustrate the use of this model, British therapists tend to confine the term social psychiatry to service activities characteristic of points "a" and "b" on the Y axis. On the other hand, for the entire (a, b, c) service range, Americans tend to prefer a series of alternative terms, especially *community psy-*

chiatry. Here social psychiatry is locked in contention with several competing labels in a sibling rivalry that thus far has defied adjustment, except in the effort of some to use the term *social and community psychiatry* as a singular noun. This fundamental split in nomenclature at the important service level has aggravated the jostled conceptual disorder.

By way of further illustration, while the British tend to use the term social psychiatry for the service section of the Y axis, Americans such as Rennie, Ruesch, Redlich, and Pepper have apparently (but not without some ambiguity) reserved the very same term primarily for the research sector (d, e, f) of the Y axis. An apparent exception is found in Alexander Leighton's book, *An Introduction to Social Psychiatry.*[8] Leighton there encompasses both the British and American positions by having social psychiatry semantically include both the service and research functions, thereby straddling the entire length of the Y asis.

In lexical history, it is not unusual for a term to become stretched too far in one content direction, or worse, in several directions simultaneously—where other more circumscribed words are already established. This can produce the speech-stopping spectacle of two competent professionals using the same term without knowing which of a number of mutually exclusive meanings the other fellow has in mind. For such a breakdown in communication, we can appropriately draw on the Book of Genesis to identify the condition as the Tower of Babel syndrome.

Bell and Spiegel[2] close their review with the dire prediction that "if a more adequate terminology is not instituted, then the term 'social psychiatry' will continue to be subject to the vagaries which we have outlined above." They call for, but do not offer such a terminology, although they express disappointment that the explorations by Leighton and associates[9] "produce many nuggets but no charting of the region."

To produce what they refer to as a chart of the region requires that we discriminate its component areas and subareas, assign each an appropriate place name, and indicate how the parts are topographically related to each other.*

It is first necessary to take a closer look at the relationship that exists between psychiatry and sociology and where they adjoin in their research functions. This has often been represented graphically by two interlocking circles on the same plane, as depicted in Figure 2.

In an earlier paper[11] I joined others in suggesting that the term social psychiatry be reserved exclusively for the above overlapping (cross-hatched) section of the two circles. I am led to withdraw that suggestion out of several considerations. There is the implication that the overlapping section is, or will develop into, one interdisciplinary field that warrants a single label. To be sure, Figure 2 shows what is in effect a top view, which facilitates such an impression. One gets a different perspective if he looks at the two circles in side view, like coins seen

---

*I shall not diminish my equal commitment to anthropology, sociology, and social psychology if I use the term "sociology" to refer to all three generically—i.e., as a synonym for the social sciences.

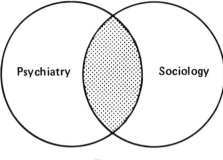

Figure 2

from their edges, as representing two parallel but separate disciplinary planes, as shown in Figure 3.

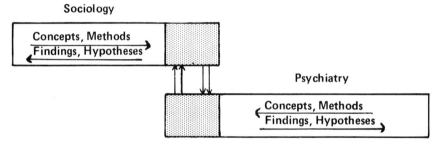

Figure 3

The point is that the overlapping section on each level is, and must remain, a subspecialty of its own parallel discipline, outfitted with that discipline's ever-evolving equipment of concepts and techniques, and replenishing the parental body of knowledge and theory with its own new data and hypotheses. To give a single label to the two overlapping sections could have the ultimate structural effect of creating a fused entity. If so, it would likely impede the vital intradisciplinary processes necessary on each plane. The vertical arrows linking the two planes in Figure 3 are meant to suggest that interdisciplinary collaboration does not require fusion.

A differentiated label is especially necessary to sustain the professional identity of social scientists specializing in the overlapping sections. Those who now have a work base in the parental discipline may find it somewhat incongruous to be assigned the mantle of what seems to be a subspecialty of another discipline. And those who work in psychiatric sites, detached from the home discipline, are often under unwitting exogenous and endogenous pressures to protectively acculturate themselves to the host discipline. For a sociologist to be identified with what appears to be a subspecialty of psychiatry tends to reinforce that pressure. To the extent that it diminishes one's identity and acuity as a social scientist, such acculturation diminishes his usefulness to *both* the parental and host disciplines. Of course, the very same considerations apply to venturous psychiatrists who have a research base in a social science department. On these grounds, I think it is essential that the two shaded areas in Figure 3 be given two separate toponymic designations.

Psychiatrists in the overlapping research sector will ultimately have to reach a consensus on their preferred name for that sector. Although not altogether satisfactory, it is didactically convenient for the time being to locate and identify that area as being more or less integral with the research sector in the three-tiered functional structure of service, training, and research within community psychiatry, as the latter is usually formulated in the United States.[1] On the other hand, as a veteran of two decades in the corresponding sector of the social science disciplines, I have found it appropriate and useful to accept designation of that sector as *psychiatric sociology*.

First, I would note that this designation is lexically coordinate with such parallel subspecialty labels as *medical sociology, educational sociology* and others in the social sciences, and with other subspecialty labels such as *psychiatric epidemiology, psychopharmacology,* and others in psychiatry.

Second, I would emphasize that identification as a psychiatric sociologist need in no way alter present patterns of affiliation and collaboration of sociologists with natural allies in the psychiatric community. Likewise the designation should not warrant the charge by psychiatrists of "empire carving" and separatism. In fact, such clarifying fission may reduce the dysfunctional identity conflicts that have long been endemic in interdisciplinary programs.

Third, it must be underscored that the term psychiatric sociology is no neologism. I will touch upon some significant points in the history of its usage. In 1955, sociologist Thomas D. Eliot called attention to a 1920 paper of his, where, in referring to the study of social aspects of psychiatric phenomena, he "coined the phrase 'psychiatric sociology' . . . as distinguishable from 'social psychiatry' which refers to *applied techniques* (Eliot's emphasis) in mental hygiene, psychiatric social work, etc." It is a pleasure to give belated acknowledgement to Professor Eliot for this contribution.

From a perusal of older textbooks however, it would appear that Eliot's coinage did not become popular in sociology until 1956. This contrasts with the considerable usage of the term social psychiatry among sociologists.[3,4] In 1956, Eliot's term was given its earliest institutional expression known to me, in the notable formation of a Committee of Psychiatric Sociology within the International Sociological Association. Led originally by the late Arnold Rose, this standing committee organized a program section at all subsequent quadrennial World Congresses of the I.S.A., including the seventh held in 1970. In 1959, the American Society for the Study of Social Problems followed by changing the name of its Social Psychiatry Committee to the Committee on Psychiatric Sociology (the sponsor of the present volume). However no comparable body is to be found within the structure of the parental American Sociological Association.

In defining the boundaries of a fledging field of knowledge, one has two choices. He can define by exclusion—by indicating where the subject begins relative to the borders of established adjoining regions. Or he can define by inclusion—by indicating what it is central, if not comprehensive. Those individuals who settle for the inclusive kind of mapping are usually satisfied to outline the core or central areas of the region and to leave precise demarcation of its ever-controversial outer boundaries to others more inclined to border warfare. To delineate community psychiatry, I first demarcate psychiatric sociology by exclusion, and then attempt to clarify its substance by outlining the topics included in its area of focus.

Three main directions of research exploration within psychiatric sociology can be seen as adjoining and coordinating with three main areas that community psychiatry, explicitly or implicitly, tends to include within its own domain. I therefore detour briefly to outline what I conclude are the three adjoining service, training, and research areas emerging under the rubric of community psychiatry. The content and coordination of the respective areas of community psychiatry and psychiatric sociology are schematically represented in Figure 4.

The goals of American community psychiatry, as embodied in the Congressional Community Mental Health Centers Act of 1963, need no repetition here. However, I would recall its key mission of coordinating and extending comprehensive mental health services to a geographically circumscribed, residential population. Its service structure seems to be taking shape in the following encompassing, tripartite form:

I.   Patient Treatment Services
    A.   The private (proprietary) sector
       1. Hospitals
       2. Clinics
       3. Office therapists
    B.   The voluntary (nonprofit) sector
       1. General hospitals
       2. Clinics
       3. Social service agencies
    C.   The public sector
       1. The long term hospital
       2. The comprehensive mental health center
          a. intramural services
          b. extramural services
       3. Social service agencies
    D.   Objective: More effective functioning of professionals, patients, and their families
II.   Group Consultation Service
    A.   Consultation to other care-giving professions

11

12

Figure 4

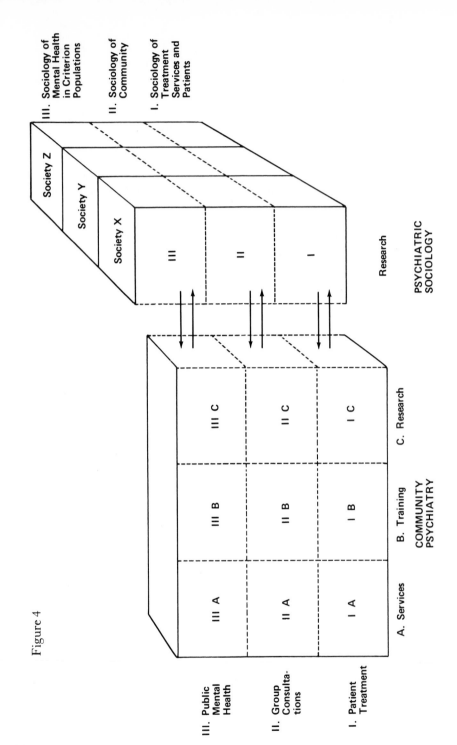

III. Sociology of Mental Health in Criterion Populations

II. Sociology of Community

I. Sociology of Treatment Services and Patients

Society Z

Society Y

Society X

III

II

I

Research

PSYCHIATRIC SOCIOLOGY

III C

II C

I C

III B

II B

I B

III A

II A

I A

A. Services

B. Training

C. Research

COMMUNITY PSYCHIATRY

III. Public Mental Health

II. Group Consultations

I. Patient Treatment

B. Consultation to "gate-keeper" persons in organized, face to face, lay groups and institutions

C. Objectives
1. Early case detection and referral
2. More effective care-giver and group functioning

III. Preventive Mental Health Services (coordinate with public health service in general medicine)
   A. Change-oriented consultation to policy making or policy influencing bodies on municipal, state, and federal levels
   B. Change-oriented consultation to educative media
   C. Objective: Prevention of illness through more effective social system functioning.

Service types I, II, and III can be seen as involving a progressively lesser degree of program organization and development. The service coverage of these three types can be schematically represented in the form of a pyramid as depicted in Figure 5 in which the vertical dimension reflects the social distance downward from the patient and his family, and the horizontal dimension reflects variations in the geographical dispersion of service coverage outward from the core treatment facilities.

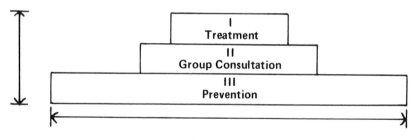

Figure 5

It is also possible to delineate three parallel research levels as the major, but not all inclusive, framework for psychiatric sociology. However, what I have selectively outlined under each level below is meant to be illustrative and suggestive, rather than comprehensive. The reader may refer back to Figure 4 for a schematic representation of these research levels.

Level I: Sociological studies of various patient traffics and of their destinations in treatment sites.
   A. The sociology of patienthood: the typology of lifetime patient-career-lines—their linear, cyclical, circular, and disjunctive movement patterns. The patient in the nonsystem maze of the treatment system.
   B. Social structure and social process involving patients and staff, in particular, kinds of service facilities and modalities, particularly the

newer types developed during the past decade. Here the series of notable studies of mental hospitals stand as models for further research.

C. The New Haven investigations[7] uncovered intrusions of social class elements that bias treatment decisions and violate professional values and goals. There has not been a corresponding research focus on intrusions of other kinds of socially structured biases into the therapeutic process, for example, racial, religious, age, and sex biases that vary independently of the social class-based attitudes of professionals.

D. Diagnostic procedures of psychiatry deal extensively with the intrapsychic realm of the patient, but are fragmentary and unsystematic with regard to his behaviors in the interpersonal domain. Social role theory is waiting to be conceptually expanded and empirically implemented in creating a typology of global interpersonal performance profiles.[12]

E. Mental health professionals form an enormously complex sociocultural community that warrants attention in its own right. Moreover, it is being buffeted about by tides of change, generated by exogenous and endogenous forces. A research program directed to this crucial theater of our embattled times has been set forth in a seminal paper by Schatzman and Strauss.[10]

F. Of special relevance to training on this level is that flux in community mental health producing acute role-retooling and conflicting professional identity problems. The new directions of community mental health are turning young psychiatrists, clinical psychologists, and psychiatric social workers from the private to the public sector, and from one-to-one relationships to milieu modalities. Rarely has sociology had the opportunities for research into professional self-remodeling on so large and rapid a scale.

Level II: Sociological studies of the community: delineation of anatomical structure and operating processes.

A. The formal structure: delineations of institutions, organizations, and
1. their constituencies
2. their leadership corps as power fulcrums
3. their action orientations and styles
4. their interdigitations.

B. The informal structure: networks of people affiliated informally outside institutions and organizations, but
1. having active or latent conduits into institutions and organizations
2. and offering untapped resources as levers for community action and change—i.e., they are nonvisible, potentially influential and powerful.

C. Individuals who are socially isolated: the nonaffiliated marginal, inert people, often the highest risk element and in need of helping services.

14

Level II of psychiatric sociology is intended to coordinate with Level II in community psychiatry, group consultation services. Its inclusion is partially prompted by the strong impression that some psychiatrists, who are leading advocates of group consultation services, reflect a limited grasp of the fact that the community is an extremely complex system with intricate depths beneath the surface level visible to the lay observer. Psychiatrists invariably think of the community mental health center as a bigger and better organized mechanism for the delivery of more effective treatment and consultation services. But they vary considerably in the extent to which they envisage and commit themselves to the involvement of a broad spectrum of community resources in developing the center, from its earliest planning stages onward.

Sociological studies of the community should enlarge the skill for making the center not only an institution in and for the community, but also of the community's making. Such research can also facilitate evaluation of the impact and penetration of community psychiatry's three-pronged service structure into the community's various population groups, institutions, and organizations. This brings us to the final sector of psychiatric sociology.

Level III: Sociological studies of mental health in general and of criterion nonpatient populations.

    A. The core of this research will continue to be epidemiological investigations designed to ferret out etiological factors associated with the whole range of mental health differences. However, more kinds of populations need study. Deeper kinds of study are required, going beneath manifest mental health differences; for example, into latent differences in immunity versus susceptibility to disorganization, and into self-management and self-evaluation functions of the ego. A large coverage of environmental factors can now be engineered in cross-sectional investigations, including the interpretation of macrosociological and microsociological family contexts.

    B. Longitudinal (life history) research is needed with a focus on:
        1. socialization processes as emergents from the properties of family and peer group organization and
        2. on the life outcome criteria of specific morbidities, longevity, and various causes of death as consequences of sociopsychological antecedents.

    C. Mental disorder is one species in a larger genus of stigmatized behavior types. The genus involves group definitions of deviancies and attempts to reverse, limit, or quarantine what are conceived of as being potentially disruptive and contagious role-contract defaults. The recent burgeoning social science literature bearing on these phenomena is significant in its promise, but research is now in order to test and refine these conceptualizations.

D. Developments in social role theory must be tested and expanded, in both general and patient populations to provide criteria for evaluation, diagnosis, and prognosis of interpersonal competence and intrapsychic resistance to social trauma.

E. We can look forward to further studies of criterion populations, for example, those who have been systematically exposed to large scale exclusions, deprivations, and punishments, such as impoverished Whites, Blacks, American Indians, and concentration camp survivors.

F. A series of national sample surveys over a period of time are indispensable if we are ever to understand the mental health consequences of long-term, and seemingly paradoxical counter-trends, as follows:
    1. Expanding affluence and persistent multigeneration poverty
    2. Rising education and shrinking environmental challenge
    3. The metropolitan polarization of mass cultural stimulation and sensory deprivation of intimate, interpersonal stimulation.
    4. Bureaucratization and dehumanization
    5. Secularism with widening horizons of freedom and shrinking moral anchorages

G. Overall, mental health in the general population is a window which gives a penetrating view to the sociologist of the interior dysfunctions of a rapidly changing social system with its surface a mixture of conflicting assets and liabilities.

The three central concerns proposed for psychiatric sociology above may be geographically extended into research in other societies. Here psychiatric sociologists join with social scientists and psychiatrists engaged in transcultural research. A current and convenient example is the investigation that I am now directing in a 500-year-old program of foster family care for patients with chronic metal illness that is based in Geel, Belgium.[13] This broad spectrum study of a natural therapeutic community is being carried out as an international, multidisciplinary collaboration between the University of Louvain and Columbia University.

The formulations presented in this chapter add up to the key suggestion that the overburdened dysfunctional term of social psychiatry be retired. This fused field label should be replaced with community psychiatry and psychiatric sociology as designations of subspecialties having separate but closely coordinated functions. This would be a step toward moving both sociology and psychiatry from a befogging dissension on nomenclature toward clarity and consensus about their shared interests and goals.

REFERENCES

1. ADELSON, D.: "Research in Community Psychiatry," in L. Bellak (ed.): *Handbook of Community Psychiatry and Community Mental Health*. New York: Grune and Stratton, 1964.
2. BELL, N., AND SPIEGEL, J.: "Social Psychiatry: Vagaries of a Term." *Archives of General Psychiatry* 14: 337-345, 1966.
3. CLAUSEN, J., AND KOHN, M.: "The Ecological Approach in Social Psychiatry." *American Journal of Sociology* 60: 140-151, 1954.
4. DUNHAM, H.: "Social Psychiatry." *American Sociological Review* 13: 183-197, 1948.
5. ELIOT, T.: "Interactions of Psychiatric and Social Theory Prior to 1940," in A. Rose (ed.): *Mental Health and Mental Disorder*. New York: Norton, 1955.
6. GOLDSTON, S.: *Concepts of Community Psychiatry*. Washington: Government Printing Office, 1965.
7. HOLLINGSHEAD, A., AND REDLICH, F.: *Social Class and Mental Illness*. New York: Wiley, 1958.
8. LEIGHTON, A.: *An Introduction to Social Psychiatry*. Springfield, Ill.: Charles C Thomas, 1960.
9. LEIGHTON, A., CLAUSEN, J., AND WILSON, R.: *Explorations in Social Psychiatry*. New York: Basic Books, 1957.
10. SCHATZMAN, L. AND STRAUSS, A.: "A Sociology of Psychiatry." *Social Problems* 14: 3-16, 1966.
11. SROLE, L.: "Selected Sociological Perspectives," in S. Goldston (ed.): *Concepts of Community Psychiatry*. Washington: Government Printing Office, 1965.
12. SROLE, L.: "Medical and Sociological Models in Assessing Mental Health," in S. Sells (ed.): *The Definition and Measurement of Mental Health*. Washington: Government Printing Office, 1968.
13. SROLE, L., AND SCHRIJVERS, J.: "Geel, Belgium: The Prototype Therapeutic Community." Paper presented to American Psychiatric Association annual meeting, Boston, 1968.
14. THEODORSON, G., AND THEODORSON, A.: *Modern Dictionary of Sociology*. New York: Crowell, 1969.
15. ZUBIN, J., AND FREYHAN, F.: *Social Psychiatry*. New York: Grune and Stratton, 1968.

Part II

THEORY AND METHOD IN PSYCHIATRIC SOCIOLOGY

INTRODUCTION

Integrating theoretical constructs and research methodology is central to the success of any scientific discipline. This integration has been particularly difficult in the social and behavioral sciences because the concepts often lack the clear-cut operational definitions necessary for empirical research. The lack of precise explanation and prediction in the behavioral sciences is reflected in the gap between concepts and their operations, compounded by a lack of consensus about definitions.

A focal issue in psychiatric sociology is the definition and measurement of the phenomena which we are attempting to study. Much theory and research is focused upon mental illness, but we lack consensus over both the conceptual and operational meanings of this term. Many sociologists have been uncomfortable in accepting the validity of psychiatric disorders as defined by psychiatry because there appears to be evidence of the biases inherent in both referral and diagnosis; nonetheless many individuals involved in research have been forced to rely on psychiatrists' labels for the delineation of study populations. For example, psychiatric referrals may reflect actual mental illness, however they may also infer that those who are *not* referred must be performing their roles with at least minimal adequacy, regardless of any psychiatric symptoms evident upon scrutiny by a field research team. Many sociologists have felt that the study of formally diagnosed cases is grossly inaccurate in terms of true epidemiology, tending to inflate rates among the segments of society more visible to the agents of social control. This has led some sociologists to develop measurements of "mental health" and "mental illness" independent of psychiatric definitions: the well-known measure of "happiness" used by Bradburn and Caplovitz[1] and the measurement of "mental health" developed by Kornhauser[7] are representative of such an approach. Such a procedure makes it difficult to compare data based on such definitions with data collected from populations formally labeled by psychiatrists. Thus, in the use of labelled populations one must sacrifice conceptual clarity for operational convenience, while in the use of independent indices one may be satisfied with his concepts but be unable to gauge the social reality reflected in his operational definitions.

The use of partial compromise to this dilemma has become increasingly popular during the past decade. It is the use of instruments which essentially mimic a psychiatric diagnosis in that they are substantially predictive of a psychiatrist's judgment of the presence of impairment.[5,6] While this approach comes closer to a legitimate epidemiological method of case finding, the results of such a strategy yield only a global definition of "impairment" rather than indexing the specific disorders used in psychiatric diagnosis. Thus while one can distinguish the impaired from the unimpaired utilizing this method, he cannot compute rates of untreated depression, schizophrenia, etc., the categories needed for comparability with psychiatric records. Furthermore, it is usually difficult to defend the cutting points used to delineate the impaired from the unimpaired segments of a sample population. Finally, while the instrument mimics a diagnosis of impairment, it does not tap the social processes which bring an individual to psychiatric attention.

These issues reflect concern about the proper relationship between psychiatric sociology and psychiatry. Some sociologists see their role as being part of the effort to improve the nature and quality of health care delivery systems while others are oriented to exposing institutional psychiatry as a discriminatory and dangerous agency of social control. Such orientations affect both the choice of research problems and the selection of methodological strategies. These pro- and anti-psychiatry orientations can be seen as polar points of a continuum, with the majority of psychiatric sociologists having ambiguous feelings about the nature and ultimate purpose of their research efforts.

With diffusion of perspectives within the field, we cannot present *the* theory of psychiatric sociology or *the* method of psychiatric sociology. Growth in interest gives no promise of increased consensus or centralized organization of research efforts in the future. It is likely, however, that scholars will give more attention in the future to the larger theoretical and methodological issues of psychiatric sociology, particularly as such issues affect relationships between sociology and psychiatry.

The four chapters in Part II reflect somewhat divergent views of the nature of psychiatric sociology and its central issues. Weinberg's chapter is based on extensive research experience in psychiatric sociology. He cogently points to dilemmas of the sociologist and the psychiatrist attempting to communicate over the issue of the causes of mental illness. As Dunham[3] has pointed out, much research in psychiatric sociology has been marked by confusion over levels of analysis, i.e., using social system level data to explain individual behavioral variation. Weinberg says that etiological explanations deserve renewed interest by contemporary psychiatric sociologists. Indirectly, his appeal is being met by the increasing attraction to ethnomethodology[2] which may be applied to etiological factors based in interaction. Weinberg's consideration of problem-centered versus theory-centered research in psychiatric sociology directly relates to the scope of work for psychiatric sociologists set forth by Srole in Chapter 1. While there is no doubt that research funding is playing a role in determining the directions of interest in psychiatric sociology, it must be recognized that studies of mental illness as well as research on psychiatric practice can contribute the answers to broader sociological questions.

The fact that sociology operates within a societal context makes variation in research emphases an expected part of the ongoing life of the field. This bears directly upon Weinberg's call for further attention to the issues of social class and schizophrenia, social isolation and schizophrenia, and cultural variations in the rates of schizophrenia and manic depression. He is correct in pointing out that previous research has yielded intriguing results that call for further empirical replication as well as theoretical expansion. Weinberg emphasizes that further study of these questions may bring these middle range theories closer to maturity; current trends however, indicate that sociologists' attention is being drawn elsewhere to problems conceived as being significant by the federal government, such as alcoholism, drug abuse, crime, and health care delivery. To take one of Weinberg's examples, it is likely that the decline of interest in the relationship between social class and schizophrenia is tied to the retreat in the War on Poverty, with the codification of existing data on this subject awaiting the attention of competent personnel who are not attracted to ongoing funding. Finally, the Weinberg chapter, as well as the previous chapter by Srole, contains elements of intellectual autobiography which are valuable in tracing the development of psychiatric sociology.

The frame of reference changes sharply with Chapter 3 on labeling theory by Fletcher, Manning, Reynolds, and Smith. These authors present the essential features of the labeling perspective applied to mental illness. They interlard their presentation with critiques of various assumptions and propositions of labeling theorists. Focusing primarily on the work of Goffman and Scheff, Fletcher and associates present the potential career phases of the individual who is labeled as mentally ill. In their criticisms a theme presented in the Srole chapter reemerges: labeling theorists have quickly drawn conclusions about the careers of the mentally ill without paying full attention to the social nature of mental illness. This indicates that labeling theory would be strengthened by the inputs of clinical psychiatry. For example, many writings couched in the labeling perspective have tended to assume that the initial events of "residual deviance" i.e., the term Scheff uses for "mentally ill" behaviors, are innocuous events which lead to the victimization of the proposed deviant. This assumption neglects the fact that although many initial symptoms are indeed dramatic, families and "significant others" often go to great lengths to normalize deviant behavior before bringing it to the attention of labeling agents. While labeling theorists tend to pose initial mental illness behaviors as benign, they seem to contradict themselves in describing the manner in which such deviants become "locked into" the mentally ill role. It is assumed that innocent persons with capricious symptoms receive a label which is socially dramatic, such as schizophrenia, as a result of the inexact processes of psychiatric diagnosis. As Gove[4] has pointed out, sweeping generalizations of labeling theory ignore the fact that many psychiatric labels are indeed reactions to aberrant and disruptive behavior which precedes the actual labeling. It is difficult however, to accept Gove's counter-assumption that psychiatric labeling is usually justifiable. The nature and effects of reactions of laymen prior to labeling are generally neglected in labeling theory formulations.

Fletcher and associates go on to criticize Goffman's conceptualization of the mental hospital, indicating that he neglects some of its crucial organizational features. They, like Gove, point out the necessity of increased attention to the mentally ill individual and his behavior as a determinant in the labeling processes rather than viewing his behavior strictly as the outcome of labeling processes.

It is important to consider the extent to which the labeling perspective can become an integral part of psychiatric sociology that is viewed as legitimate by social psychiatrists. The extent to which writings within the labeling perspective have been couched as broadsides against the practice of psychiatry accounts for the apparent rejection of this perspective by social psychiatrists, with the notable exceptions of Szasz, Leifer, Laing, and Cooper. The labeling perspective has generated considerable enthusiasm within the field of sociology and may in large part account for the renewed interest in the sociology of deviance. It is likely however, that the "deviant as a victim" emphasis that has pervaded many of the labelists' writings has created a defensiveness on the part of psychiatry and other disciplines of social control that may be difficult to overcome. As Fletcher and associates demonstrate, the labeling perspective may be enhanced by the interdisciplinary involvement of social psychiatrists in its further explorations. But will psychiatrists advance efforts which they perceive as indictments of their profession and as being contrary to their own interests?

In Chapters 4 and 5 issues of methodology are the concern. In Chapter 4, Robins is primarily concerned with how the etiology of psychiatric disorder can be established through field research designs. While the assumptions underlying her presentation contrast sharply with the assumptions of labeling theory, she clearly illustrates how research on psychiatric disorders highlights basic dilemmas in social research methods. Despite improvements in case-findings where researchers have access to epidemiological resources as central case registers (in contrast to research where case definition is limited to those hospitalized in public facilities), research designs still largely neglect the temporal dimensions that are crucial in determining causation.

Unlike many psychiatric sociologists, Robins recognizes that competing explanations of causation, such as those based on genetics, must be taken into account in the most sophisticated sociological design. She outlines suggestions for longitudinal designs which approximate a natural experiment, giving the researcher further control in establishing causation. Robins deals directly with the question of the dependent variable in research in psychiatric sociology. As one whose extensive research experience has been primarily in a psychiatric setting, she implies the need to focus upon discrete disorders, advocating research efforts where results can be generalized to the nosological categories employed in psychiatry.

In contrast to most labeling theorists, Robins takes psychiatric definitions as givens and then outlines how the methods of social research can be employed to explain the existence of such behaviors. Such a position accepts the reality of psychiatry as a functioning social institution. Etiological studies which employ psychiatric definitions in delineating research populations can provide valuable insights into the operation of psychiatry. Thus Robins' chapter comprises an excellent blueprint for rigorous research on the developmental course of psychiatric disorders which can be fruitfully combined with the richness of theoretical perspectives such as the labeling orientation.

Safilios-Rothschild and Moore explore basic strategies in cross-national comparative research in psychiatric sociology. Much of the existing literature is focused soley on data generated in America. An international perspective is called for in Srole's research program and specifically illustrated in Weinberg's studies of manic-depressive psychoses. Safilios-Rothschild and Moore focus on the issues surrounding the role of the outsider which the researcher, who is attempting to study psychiatric phenomena in a culture other than his own, will encounter. Such problems are likewise encountered in a range of research situations where the researcher is an outsider, such as in the mental hospital, albeit to a lesser degree. They deal with such ways and means issues as obtaining cooperation and developing a research staff in the host culture, constructing instruments which can be generalized across cultures, and going about the actual processes of data collection. They focus in on a range of methodological issues surrounding the comparability of data which they aptly phrase "the crux of the matter."

This chapter places strong emphasis on the necessity of close cooperation between the sociologist and the psychiatrist. The psychiatric sociologist working in another culture cannot proceed in his research with the autonomy that may be possible in his own culture. He is, instead, heavily dependent on native psychiatrists both for access to research subjects and for an understanding of the culture's systems of diagnosis and treatment as well as for its definitions of deviance. Safilios-Rothschild and Moore clearly illustrate that the cross-cultural research design may provide a model for interdisciplinary cooperation that has, in a large part, been lacking in research conducted within the boundaries of the United States.

Taken together, these chapters provide several general insights. On the one hand they demonstrate the lack of consensus within psychiatric sociology about what constitutes significant theoretical problems, but there appears to be a consensus over the methodological strategy needed for theory construction in psychiatric sociology. The chapters demonstrate that the gulf between traditional research and emerging perspectives such as labeling need not be as wide as one might think. The chapters highlight the need for sociologists to better understand psychiatry and make further attempts at interdisciplinary endeavors despite the implicit barriers to such strategies.

REFERENCES

1. BRADBURN, N., AND CAPLOVITZ, D.: *Reports on Happiness.* Chicago: Aldine, 1965.
2. DOUGLAS, J. (ed.): *Understanding Everyday Life.* Chicago: Aldine, 1970.
3. DURHAM, H. W.: "Anomie and Mental Disorder," in M. B. Clinard (ed.): *Anomie and Deviant Behavior.* New York: The Free Press, 1964.
4. GOVE, W. R.: "Societal Reaction as an Explanation of Mental Illness." *American Sociological Review* 35: 873-884, 1970.
5. LANGNER, T. S.: "The Twenty-Two Item Index of Psychiatric Impairment." *Journal of Health and Human Behavior* 4: 269-274, 1962.
6. LEIGHTON, D. C. et al.: *The Character of Danger.* New York: Basic Books, 1963.
7. KORNHAUSER, A.: *Mental Health of the Industrial Worker.* New York: John Wiley, 1965.

CHAPTER 2

Issues in the Scope and Theory of Psychiatric Sociology

S. KIRSON WEINBERG

Issues of approach and selected issues of content in psychiatric sociology are the subjects of this chapter. The issues of approach include the scope, direction, and continuity of theory in this field. The issues of content cover the logically-derived as well as the unsettled empirical hypotheses. The issues of approach have arisen because of the indefinite area of convergence between psychiatry and sociology. Psychiatrists have acknowledged that there are sociocultural, as well as psychological and biological, influences upon disordered behavior. Sociologists have expanded their theories and techniques to include the study of disordered behavior. Since each discipline has adapted this area to its speciality, different blends of psychiatry and sociology have developed which affect the scope and continuity of theory. Likewise, action implications of the study of disordered behavior raise issues of concern.

Within the field of sociology itself, there are divergent emphases concerning the proper scope of inquiry to be focused on disordered behavior. Should the scope of inquiry be limited to the epidemiological correlates and cultural variations in disordered behavior, or should it include the social etiology of persons with disordered behavior? From another position, should the study of disordered behavior be limited to the social definitions and reactions to it and the search for social etiology be abandoned? These issues in psychiatric sociology are representative of the reflections and extensions of basic disagreement among sociologists concerning the scope and depth of sociology itself.

The scope of psychiatric sociology varies too with the definition of disordered behavior. Within a sociopsychological context, disordered behavior is an extreme and incapacitating form of disorganized behavior. It differs from the psychiatric term of *mental illness* that confuses the word mental with the social personality, connoting a *functional illness* as being parallel to an *organic illness.* Actually the term *personality disorders* would be preferable but this concept already has a specialized connotation of acting out or sociopathic disorders. Disordered behavior as defined here includes 1) personality or *functional* psychoses, such as schizophrenia, manic-depression, and paranoia, 2) neuroses, and 3) sociopathy. It represents one type of deviant behavior; many individuals who fall into these categories depart from established patterns of behavior and are defined as being deviant. Thus, most individuals with psychotic disorders would be considered deviant with the exception of some paranoiacs who when capable of functioning in certain independent roles might not be so defined. Some neurotic patients who exhibit manifestly bizarre or norm-violating behavior would be considered deviant; other neurotic individuals who inhibit exposure of their conflicts would be regarded as being socially normal. Since sociopaths are troublesome and get into recurrent difficulties, their behavior is usually defined as being deviant.

One point of view in psychiatric sociology would limit its scope to the social aspects of the development, treatment, and prevention of these forms of disordered behavior on the assumption that they might have a social etiology. Another would extend psychiatric sociology to include the degree of social correlation between organic disorders such as paresis or cerebral arteriosclerosis, while a third would deal with the learned forms of deviance such as juvenile delinquency, adult crime, alcoholism, prostitution, and drug addiction. A fourth omnibus position espoused by psychiatrists would encompass the study of the social aspects of all types of behavior.

Issues of content focused upon in this chapter involve mainly analyses of schizophrenia, and, to a lesser extent, manic-depressive illness. Research on both of these types of psychoses has developed a great many generalizations and interpretations, some of which are inconclusive and the focus of disagreement. These issues include epidemiological distributions, prevalence in cross-cultural variations, and the influences of interpersonal etiology.

The problems in psychiatric sociology which I shall discuss include: 1) the scope of psychiatric sociology, 2) theoretical schemes and research problems, 3) problem-centered and theory-centered research, 4) selected substantive issues, 5) social relations, isolation, and schizophrenia, and 6) the onset of schizophrenia and manic-depressive psychoses in different cultures.

THE SCOPE OF PSYCHIATRIC SOCIOLOGY

Psychiatric sociology has emerged from two disciplines with different perspectives and goals. It has developed in part from psychiatry, which is an applied, eclectic, multidimensional field as well as a healing science and a means of psychotherapeutic engineering. In perspective, theory, and method, it has developed from sociology which is a specialized, unidimensional research discipline with a consistent body of theory. As an uneasy progeny of these parent fields, the nature and scope of psychiatric sociology remains the basis for disagreement.

The position of social psychiatry emphasizes an eclectic specialty with a multidimensional subject matter and an action oriented goal. It attempts to discover a correlation between biological, psychological, and social variables which contribute to mental disorders. It frequently directs the results of its findings as means to improve the techniques relevant to the psychotherapy, rehabilitation, or prevention of disordered behavior. This multidisciplinary view, expounded by Rennie[29] and Ruesch,[31] presents social psychiatry as a coordinating field of the social and psychological sciences, which utilizes the findings of several of the behavioral sciences for understanding, treating, and preventing disordered behavior.

A somewhat restricted but consistent approach to these phenomena is psychiatric sociology. Its assumptions, theories, and methods are of a sociological nature, while its subject matter has traditionally been within the scope of psychiatry; it focuses on the social aspects of disordered behavior. This position would logically consign studies of the correlation between social and biological aspects of disordered behavior to medical sociology and in this way achieve a theoretical consistency. Through concerted scientific scrutiny, psychiatric sociologists aspire to attain a body of logically related and empirically-validated set of generalizations concerning the social facets of the development, care, treatment, and prevention of disordered behavior.[42]

These divergent approaches to the study of the social aspects of mental disorders, whether or not in frontal disagreement, imply different research goals, problems, and roles for the sociologist. In social psychiatry the collaborative inquiry of both disciplines ideally results in a coordination of two frames of reference. This usually involves a division of labor in which the psychiatrist ascertains diagnostic types and case populations to be studied, while the sociologist (who may devise the research design) relates sociological and demographic variables to variations within the population under study. From this collaborative approach to research, important epidemiological findings have emerged. For example, social psychiatric research conducted within an epidemiological framework has generated considerable knowledge about the distribution of specified mental disorders in socioeconomic structures.[45]

A crucial impasse in the use of this approach arises, however, when efforts are made to employ these epidemiological findings as indicators of the breakdown of the socialized person within a sociocultural context. Although some distributions have been interpreted on the sociocultural level, other analyses have been interpreted on more individualistic terms. For example, the concentration of cases of schizophrenia in the lower socioeconomic stratum may be interpreted as a consequence of the stresses indigenous to this particular stratum, or as the result of the downward social drift of schizophrenics into this stratum. When, however, social mobility is analyzed in terms of its effect on the socialized person, epidemiological data have been used to infer psychoanalytic, genetic, or other individualistic processes rather than to indicate social psychological processes.[33] This recourse to dual frames of reference is understandable when one deals with the social correlation between biological or biophysical phenomena. It becomes less admissible, however, when it becomes evident that some disorders may be influenced etiologically by social or sociopsychological processes; nonetheless, this problem has been disregarded in much sociological inquiry. A methodological assumption which has led to the circumvention of this potential etiological continuity between social indicators and social processes is that sociology as a science should be concerned with ascertaining accurate correlations per se, without attempting an extrapolative interpretation or explanation.

By contrast, the psychiatric sociologist who analyzes disordered behavior as social phenomena interprets epidemiological distributions in the socioeconomic structure, or interprets varying organizations of mental hospitals in terms of the socialized person functioning in a series of social structures and not as an isolated organism or reactive system. It is obvious, therefore, that research probing should aim to ferret out the social processes reflected in and indicated by the epidemiological distributions.

The study of psychiatric sociology in terms of this integral view of disordered behavior is hindered by constraints from outside as well as inside the discipline. The clinician frequently regards the sociologist's interest in the personality development of disordered behavior as an intrusion into the area of diagnostics, and away from his effective research role. For example, the sociologist has been discouraged from conducting developmental studies. This has resulted from the fact that frequently the sociologist lacks access to clinical data and subjects, and that his research must begin with a psychiatric diagnosis which is formulated from a psychiatric frame of reference. As a result, the sociologist is often thrust into a kind of adjunct research role.

Within the field of sociology itself, two recent shifts in approach have complicated the type of psychiatric sociology previously described. One general shift in sociology has been away from the study of the socialization of personality to a concern with social behavior in terms of social organization, social stratification, and acculturation to subcultures. In fact, the term *socialization* has been interpreted as meaning incorporation into the group as a social parallel to acculturation rather than as developmental changes that take place within the personality.[21] This shift in the emphasis of socialization and disregard of the social personality has also been noted in studies of criminal and other forms of deviant behavior which deal mainly with the influence of cultural pressures upon behavior.[42]

Another digression in psychiatric sociology has been the position, however arbitrary, that the study of the etiology of deviant behavior (of which disordered behavior is one form) is obsolete and that a more appropriate concern is with the consequences, reactions, and societal definitions of deviant behavior.[20] Individuals subscribing to this position, although acknowledging epidemiology as a legitimate concern, deliberately or inadvertently might disregard a vital part of the accrued sociological knowledge of the probable etiology of disordered behavior. Its acceptance could result in the abandonment of fruitful clues and contributions, such as the significant influences of peer relations, of work activity, of marital relations, and of social isolation upon certain types of disordered behavior, especially upon schizophrenia. Restricting the study of disordered behavior to societal definitions and reactions is viewed as an integral aspect of the symbolic interactionist school of thought. Although the symbolic designation of objects, persons, and types is within the symbolic interactionist position, symbolic interaction itself also is concerned with the causal development and career of behavioral trends and patterns acquired from an individual's orbit of social relationships.[25, 30, 39]

The scope of psychiatric sociology then narrows down to two issues. The first involves social psychiatry as opposed to psychiatric sociology, or the development of a multidimensional, eclectic, bio-psychosociological position as opposed to a unidimensional, consistent, sociological, and sociopsychological approach. The second issue deals with the controversy over a continuing concern with social etiology leading to and explaining social breakdown, and leading to the societal definitions of disordered behavior. This viewpoint is opposed to a scope limited chiefly to the study of societal definitions of, and reactions to, types of people with disordered behavior.

THEORETICAL SCHEMES AND RESEARCH PROBLEMS

By its assumptions, theoretical scheme influences the selection of problems for study. Since the psychogenic view of personality has predominated as an interpretation of the etiology of disordered behavior, most developmental studies by non-Freudians as well as Freudians have been concerned with the influence of the family upon infancy and childhood. Comparatively few studies have dealt with subsequent periods of life or with associations and groups other than the family. The upsurge of attention to adult socialization[4] reflects the sociological position which maintains that personality structure is not necessarily fixed in early life; hence early experience may not be completely explanatory of subsequent disordered behavior. This position has provided the rationale for investigations by psychiatric sociologists on the influence of the peer group, school, work, and marital situations upon disordered behavior. Examples include studies of disordered behavior among combat soldiers, which indicate that relatively stable persons experience neurotic and psychotic breakdowns during severe combat stress.[8, 15, 38]

The research autonomy of the psychiatric sociologist in terms of his theoretical position has not been fully expressed. Because the sociologist is often a research adjunct to the clinician, the clinician frequently selects the topic and direction of the social psychiatric inquiry. Consequently, the study of the person with disordered behavior from the sociological view has not been allowed to run its logical course, and as a result has been largely confined to epidemiological indicators of the social processes contributing to disordered behavior.

On another level, the sociological version of disordered behavior has influenced a shift from the study of hospitalized psychotics to the study of individuals in terms of their degrees of stability as they function in the community. It paved the way for the Midtown Manhattan Study, in which a general population has been analyzed in terms of degree of social stability.[35] The standard of stability in the general population has been revised from a clinically ideal norm to an empirically gauged—if clinical—reality. Consequently, the study of the differences between the nonhospitalized person and the hospitalized person has been revised to one of degree from one of kind.

This sociological position differs from another sociological view which confuses normal behavior in the community with personal stability. This view gives credence to the insanity-sanity dichotomy, which holds that only treated or hospitalized persons are abnormal and those outside this realm are normal. But as is increasingly evident, socially vulnerable persons, such as the poor and racial minorities, are more apt to be committed to a state mental hospital than those from the middle class majorities. The Midtown Manhattan Study used clinical criteria which could readily be translated into a patient's degree of ego strength and tolerance for adversity. Its findings indicated that a person does not have to be emotionally stable to participate in this urban community and can remain socially normal. This means that the community definition of normal is not equivalent with personal emotional stability. Many socially normal persons were found to be emotionally impaired or incapacitated as a result of severe conflict.

The Midtown Manhattan Study represented the use of an innovative sociological approach in psychiatric sociology. But its methods did not reveal in what ways the impaired or incapacitated individuals were hindered in their social roles and participation in comparison to those inhabitants who were symptom free. In this sense, this study was static and clinical rather than dynamic and sociopsychological. Furthermore, the implication of a homogenized socially defined normality implies that people who fall into this criteria are broadly similar in their life experiences and in the ways they internalize and react to their experiences. Actually, only a small visible segment of a person's behavior can be socially defined because much of what occurs in private life remains opaque to human gaze and judgment. Study of the diversified inner organization of personality would reveal varying degrees of tolerance for routine duties and for challenging complexities. The Midtown Manhattan Study can be credited with making a start in this direction by demonstrating that varying degrees of instability or stability can be detected among persons defined as being normal in a heterogeneous and highly urbanized community. Nonetheless, from a developmental perspective, personal stability reflects the influences of one's social milieu and should be so studied.

Another issue arises from this viewpoint and concerns the locus of disordered behavior. The nominalistic or individualistic view regards the etiological locus of the disorder to reside mainly in the individual's inherent traits and personality predispositions. This basis for disorder is sought within the organization of personality traits. By contrast, the sociologist's realistic or interactionist view, when logically pursued, regards the person with disordered behavior as an emergent of the social situations and groups in which he participates. Consequently, the amount of stress present in these situations, groups, and social relations would be considered the loci which contribute to the individual's eventual disordered behavior. The person is then viewed primarily as a product of influences by a hostile and demeaning person or group, whether this be a parent, sibling, peer, teacher, or institution. Evidence of this influence is present in the children of pathological parents; among withdrawn youths who have been rejected by their peers; in a distressed wife who is a victim of a domineering husband; among hospitalized patients who are agitated as a result of conflicts between staff; and among some patients immobilized by chronic schizophrenia in mental hospitals whose apathy may reflect the institutional demands of hospital policy rather than their psychological condition.

Thus, the issue is drawn between the etiological loci, or an individual's genetic or psychogenetic disposition, and a focus on stresses present during and after early childhood which reflect the pathology located in social roles, groups, and other relationships of the afflicted person. One reconciling sociological view of the loci of disorder emphasizes stress situations integrally combined with the residual traits and symptoms acquired from past experiences.

Problem-Centered and Theory-Centered Research

The type of direction and degree of continuity of theory in psychiatric sociology are contingent upon the alternative approaches of problem-centered and theory-centered research. From the problem-centered approach the investigator selects topics for study which are considered significant by agencies, administrators, and pressure groups within the community. Since these problems shift with community needs and problems, theory-building becomes discontinuous and even chaotic with the accretion of knowledge in the field. During different periods problems have been studied by psychiatric sociologists because they are timely from a community point of view: war casualties, the mental hospital, socioeconomic status and disordered behavior, drug addiction, and community psychiatry. Frequently the findings of these studies have been oriented toward social action with subsidiary attention to theory-building. Thus, some problems are investigated intensively and then abandoned in favor of other urgent problems because of shifting community pressures and selective subsidies allocated for investigating the new problems. As a result many theoretical problems are left dangling and remain unresolved. However, some research on such topics as socioeconomic status, mobility and schizophrenia, cultural complexity and schizophrenia, or the role of isolation in the etiology of schizophrenia have been objects of persistent inquiry, representing a pursuit of the theory-centered approach. The fact remains, however, that the continuity of research depends in part upon the selection of research problems for community subsidy and support.

The theory-centered approach is concerned with problems that arise from knowledge gaps within psychiatric sociology. It selects certain topics for inquiry because of inconclusive or incomplete findings in these areas. Its aims are essentially scientific; it tries to verify tenuous generalizations and thereby pursues theory-building in a continuous direction. This theory-centered position is inner-directed and concerned with problems in terms of scientific criteria. By contrast, the problem-centered position is directed outward, selecting problems which have community importance and which add knowledge that can be implemented into social action. Although they oppose one another in their criteria for selection of research topics, these approaches do not necessarily contradict each other in practice. Broad research problems which have been subsidized to further understanding for community action may have theoretical pertinence, such as the effects of socioeconomic status or mobility upon disordered behavior or, as in the past, effects of the mode of hospital organization upon the personality reorganization among persons with behavior disorders. The development of a theoretical framework operates within and is influenced by a sociopolitical context; full analyses of these processes is the domain of the sociology of knowledge. But this kind of introspection is vital in determining the direction of psychiatric sociology, as well as other subfields and theories in sociology.

Selected Substantive Issues in Psychiatric Sociology

Since the problem-oriented approach has been and remains ascendant in the research of psychiatric sociology, it follows that few generalizations in this specialty have achieved conclusive empirical validation. Perhaps the initial findings of the ecological distribution of schizophrenia and manic-depressive psychosis in the unplanned or laissez-faire American urban community, or the findings concerning the inverse relationship that exists between socioeconomic status and schizophrenia would have the widest consensus. The latter generalization, however, is qualified by some studies that find no such relationship and by studies that indicate that incidences of schizophrenia are concentrated in the lower classes and may not differ significantly among the other strata.

This leads to a specific substantive issue of theory in psychiatric sociology. The relationships that exist between socioeconomic status, social mobility, and schizophrenia constitute perhaps the most extensively investigated subject in the field. The varying explanations of these relationships point to a generic issue between social selection and contemporary or sequential stress as alternative explanations of the development and onset of this psychotic disorder. The controversy, however, resides in the alternatives between genetic-constitutional and psychogenetic factors—i.e., the inherent and the early-acquired predisposition to this disorder, and the varied experience of subsequent stress. Either of these situations, or very likely both, have etiological significance for the onset of this disorder, even assuming a constancy of societal definition. The concentration of higher rates of schizophrenia among members of the lower classes may result from social selection directed by defective hereditary and/or congenital traits and/or the psychogenic influence of modes of early childhood rearing within the lower strata.[6] Schizophrenia may then be a consequence of the stresses which arise from:

1. Mother-child relations.
2. Father-child relations.
3. Sibling relationships.
4. Peer relations.
5. Social relations with the opposite sex.
6. School relations and school performance.
7. Work relations and performance.
8. Marital relations.
9. Neighbor and secondary relations.
10. Shifting demands and the changes created by new age-roles in the life cycle and the facility with which one can readapt to new relationships and responsibilities.

Although the Midtown Manhattan and other studies found downwardly mobile persons to be less stable than their upward counterparts, it has not been determined to what extent downward mobility is a decisive stress factor.[36] The generic issue concerns the polarity between social selection and the sequence of stresses which may indicate alternative or combined conditions contributing to schizophrenia. This problem has not been resolved because these influences, as single and independent variables, may not explain all cases of schizophrenia. Initially, this controversy pertained to the interpretations of the urban-ecological distribution of schizophrenia. Did high rates of schizophrenia in certain communities result from stresses in the community or from the downward drift by persons predisposed to schizophrenia? In categorizing cases of schizophrenia by age, Faris and Dunham[12] found that young individuals diagnosed as being schizophrenic, for example, the catatonic types, had been long-time residents of family slum areas where they broke down and hence were possibly victimized products of the area. Paranoid individuals who had broken down in rooming house areas, however, may have not skidded downward, but rather moved in from other areas. The stresses in these highly-mobile, poverty-ridden anonymous areas hastened the psychotic onset of some residents.

Lapouse and associates[18] found that hospitalized schizophrenic patients, who were first time admissions, were residents of the area where they broke down and were not downward drifters. Redlich and Hollingshead,[28] and Tietze and associates,[37] have reported that schizophrenics in Class V have been predominantly in this class before the breakdown. Lystad,[24] however, reported that individuals suffering from schizophrenia were more downwardly mobile than were a control group of nonschizophrenics. Morris,[26] in his study of schizophrenics in England, found that they were predominantly in the lower classes while their fathers were randomly distributed through all classes. He interpreted their downward mobility as a drop rather than a drift. Dunham and his associates[9] derived similar findings.

Do stresses that exist within the lower class contribute to the higher incidence of schizophrenia, or are these persons genetically predisposed, or do they become predisposed psychogenetically? If the culture of poverty is schizophrenogenic with its pervasive social and family disorganization, modes of child rearing and modes of interpersonal relations as well as physical deprivations create stressful conditions. This can be determined more clearly by developmental studies of samples of schizophrenics in the lower social strata and other strata whether using occupation and education criteria only and/or the community criterion as well.[42]

A second substantive issue centers on social isolation and its relation to schizophrenia and other disorders. One crucial influence in the development of schizophrenia appears to be the modes of interpersonal relations and the degree of isolation experienced by the individual. Regardless of social strata, subjects who eventually become schizophrenic experience somewhat similar social relations with the mother and peers and many have been socially isolated before their breakdowns. On the interactional level, one significant issue pertains to the effects of social isolation upon schizophrenia as well as other disorders. Although several studies deal with this phenomenon, the literature generally is scant, and the knowledge concerning the effect of this variable upon schizophrenia and other disorders remains inconclusive. Operational definitions of isolation have varied from that of diminished social contacts in a community,[16] to the relative absence of peer relations,[11, 4] to my view which is withdrawal from rejection by peers of the same and opposite sex and the ensuing diffidence in renewing or pursuing these relations.[40, 42, 43] But finding that schizophrenics experience isolation from peers does not explain how isolation contributes to the disorder. I have found that some college students who have been isolated from their peers did not feel that they needed clinical help and appeared relatively stable when they were employed. Some of them had been residentially mobile so that their isolation was situational. I have also found some incidence of schizophrenia during adolescence in patients who have not been isolated from their peers. Finally, my research has disclosed some schizophrenic individuals who sustained an emotionally withdrawn attitude from childhood and intensified their isolation during adolescence.

34

From observations of these varied sequences of isolation, the issue appears to be one of identifying manifest symptoms resulting from isolation in one type of schizophrenic as compared with another who may have had friends but who broke down after a sequence of severe stress experiences. The important considerations are the impact of the type of isolation upon the individual and his manner of incorporating interpersonal experiences, or adjusting to his lack of them. Schizophrenics who have not been isolated from their peers and others before their breakdowns might be studied to determine to what extent social isolation contributed to the breakdown experience. Different variables may have similar consequences for the person with disordered behavior because there is no one-to-one relationship that exists between objective conditions and subjective reactions, such as social isolation and emotional withdrawal. From my research on this problem, isolation as a consequence of rejection involving diminution of self-worth is more destructive than is the total lack of social contacts; however, the latter situation may give rise to a feeling of imbalance in the self by creating an inability to see oneself from the perspective of a close associate.[40, 44] Thus, the isolated person may be diminished in his capacity to share perspectives for close empathic role-taking. This may lead to further withdrawal but it may not necessarily eventuate into schizophrenia. On the other hand, social isolation as a mechanism of withdrawal from initial social rejection and the apprehension of further rejection becomes a defensive posture.

Thus, the problem of how and in what manner isolation contributes to schizophrenia and to other mental disorders depends upon the type of isolation to which one is referring. The conception of the type of isolation must be clarified and its effects upon diverse categories of disordered behaviors empirically verified. Of cardinal concern is the impact of isolation on self-esteem and upon the individual's capacity to initiate, renew, and sustain his social relations. Neurotic persons may withdraw socially as a result of rejection but remain non-hallucinatory and nondelusional.[22, 23, 38] Seemingly, the effects of social rejection are not as severe among individuals with neuroses as among those who become schizophrenic. Thus, the subjective meaning of isolation and the defensive systems evolved to protect self-esteem become crucial in understanding the effects of this pathological lack of social relations.

CULTURAL VARIATIONS IN THE ONSET OF SCHIZOPHRENIA AND MANIC-DEPRESSION

A broad macrocultural issue in psychiatric sociology concerns the influence of culture complexity upon schizophrenia and manic-depressive psychosis. Complex urban culture presumably contributes to the rise in numbers of cases of schizophrenia. This hypothesis implies an inverse sociocentrism; the simple society is, for some reason, considered the healthy society. Old line field investigators including E. Faris,[10] Seligman,[34] Carothers,[3] and Devereux[5] claimed that incidence of schizophrenia was rare or did not exist in nonliterate societies isolated from Western influences. This Rousseauean approach to the nonliterate person was not without bias in obscuring a concerted search for evidence of schizophrenic behavior in these societies. E. Faris believed that the personality, as a subjective aspect of culture, would not become socially withdrawn in a society dominated by primary relations. Devereux felt that in a simple homogeneous society with a "one-answer universe" ideology, deviant versions of the culture would rarely arise.

Dhunjiboy[7] and Sachs[32] indicated that in nonliterate societies influenced by Western culture cases of schizophrenia had in fact emerged. Kardiner[17] made similar observations and claimed that schizophrenia appears transculturally because it is basically a biogenetic psychosis. Nielsen and Thompson[27] also maintained that schizophrenia is known among all cultures. Benedict and Jacks[2] also reported that investigators of nonliterate societies have observed manifestations of schizophrenia.

Field,[13] in a study of rural Ghana, observed incidence of simple schizophrenia in the most removed and isolated villages. My own inquiries in Ghana confirmed Field's findings. I found that even in the simplest village in Ghana, divergent modes of interpersonal relations ensued and that the inhabitants in vulnerable roles were likely to be abused, exploited, and exposed to intense personal strain. Some of these individuals became schizophrenic.[41]

When viewed against this background, the widely quoted study by Goldhamer and Marshall[14] of the comparative incidence of psychoses, including schizophrenia, between the 19th and the 20th centuries seems strange. They strived to test the conviction that a civilization with high degree of individuation, personal insecurity, competitiveness, and a "killing pace" was responsible for a large measure of psychotic breakdown. This hypothesis, however, was not derived from empirical inquiry, but from an untested impression. Since modes of societal definition of psychoses were roughly similar in the two historic periods, it is not surprising that rates of psychoses were similar.

Despite qualifications, severe social stress can permeate a simple society. Beaglehole[1] has differentiated between cultural and subjective complexity. A person in a very technologically complicated and culturally diverse society who leads a consistent routine may be relatively free of conflicts and threatening situations. A member of a simple culture confronted by fretful relations or conflicting situations with threatening alternatives could become severely disturbed.

Basic stresses in simple societies arise from hostile interpersonal relations whether between mother and child, peers, siblings, mates, or adult villagers. These hostilities are often expressed through witch craft and black magic. When schizophrenia is manifest in a nonliterate society, the afflicted person is not necessarily biogenetically predisposed to the psychosis. The fact that cases of schizophrenia occur in simple societies has been used by some as evidence that the disorder stems from a genetically vulnerable personality. Such reasoning is based on a misunderstanding of the meaning of homogeneous culture in nonliterate and folk societies. The norms governing behavior in such cultures, no matter how consistent, permit a wide range of responses in terms of role performances and interpersonal relations. Thus, a mother's hostility toward her child, strained marital relations, and quarrels between friends are all behaviors within the bounds of cultural acceptability. Even in the simplest society, interpersonal conflict can have traumatic effects on the interactant who is in the more vulnerable position. Despite the simplicity of the Navaho culture, Leighton and Kluckhohn[19] reported that Navaho children experience personality difficulties similar to those experienced by White American children. They attribute these difficulties to "the interpersonal relations of the groups in which the child is a member."

Cultural complexity affects individuals suffering from manic-depressive psychosis differently than it does those suffering from schizophrenia. First, incidences of schizophrenia tend to concentrate among the lower urban strata. Manic-depressive illness, especially the depressed type, does not show this concentrated pattern among the lower classes nor does it seem to be a direct outcome of urbanization; it tends instead to be associated with the middle and upper classes. Second, manic-depressive illness has been associated with technologically advanced peoples in contrast to those who are technologically underdeveloped. Thus Blacks in the rural south of the United States and the inhabitants of rural areas still under colonial domination have been imputed to have low rates of manic-depressive illness, especially the depressive type. Likewise inhabitants in several countries of sub-Sahara Africa have been found to have very low rates of manic-depressive illness, especially of the depressive type. Carothers[3] reported that only 24 or 1.6 per cent of 1508 patients in Kenya, East Africa, were diagnosed as suffering from a form of manic-depressive psychosis. Laubscher[46] found that only 3.8 per cent of 554 patients in South Africa were manic-depressive. Asuni reported in a Nigerian study that depression was infrequent and suicide, which is associated with depression, was calculated at one per 100,000 persons of the general population. Dembowitz and Carothers[47] were impressed by the rarity of depression among West African soldiers.

On the other hand, Aubin[48] reported that depression was frequent among West African soldiers. Tooth[49] reported that about 20 per cent of 178 patients examined in Ghana were manic-depressive and 2.3 per cent were of the depressive type. Field,[13] who observed the Ghanian people in their villages and shrines as well as in the mental hospital, reported that depression "was the commonest mental illness of rural women and all such women come to the shrines with self-accusations of witchcraft."

My analysis of 108 records in the State Mental Hospital in Accra indicates that 34.3 per cent of these patients had some manic or depressive symptoms, of whom 11.2 per cent were diagnosed as having depressive features. In addition, the Ghana Health Ministry reported a corrected rate of 20.8 attempted suicides per 100,000 persons 15 years of age and older.

These inconsistent rates and observations of manic-depressive psychosis, particularly the depressive type, in different sub-Sahara countries makes one suspect that a combination of the following influences have contributed to these differences:

First, psychiatrists in the sub-Sahara countries of Kenya, South Africa, Nyasaland, and Ghana limited their studies to hospitalized patients who were presumably dangerous and troublesome to the community. Since many individuals with manic-depressive psychosis conform socially, they might be underrepresented among the commitments. I found in the State Mental Hospital of Ghana that even among socially troublesome patients only about 25 per cent had depressive or manic symptoms. Field has observed that many individuals with the depressive type were not hospitalized but visited shrines to invoke the gods for help in their personal problems.

Second, psychiatrists in these sub-Sahara countries were European and based their diagnoses of manic-depression upon European models. Their focus of attention was upon similarities rather than the differences in the manifestations of depression between Europeans and sub-Sahara Africans. As a consequence, they slighted or overlooked the diverse expressions of depression among sub-Saharan patients.

Third, some psychiatrists in these hospitals were ideologically biased in their diagnoses of depression. They believed that depression was scarce among Blacks because of their "racial temperament," the technological underdevelopment of their countries, and their low socioeconomic status. Other psychiatrists such as those in Ghana, however, were not biased in their diagnoses by these social criteria.

Fourth, sociocultural influences may be the significant issues in the development of depression. Specifically, do cultures in these sub-Saharan countries fashion the self-system and guilt reaction of their inhabitants in a manner which would create or avoid severe depression? Do people in these societies externalize their aggressions and avoid self-blame? Such personality formation would clearly affect the self-control of the population and the very social control of the society. It is obvious that basic personality organization is central to this problem.

Kardiner,[17] in his analysis of the Alorese personality, reported that because of the Alorese mode of child rearing, the child did not identify with the mother, did not internalize her norms, and did not internalize aggression patterns. As a consequence, he maintained that the "child's aggressions against the mother did not ricochet back on the child in masochistic form." For this reason, he argued, "There is no depression and no suicide among the Alorese." But as a people, the Alorese were not readily amenable to social control nor could they readily control their aggressions.

Among the Gas, Ashantis, and Ewes in Ghana, as well as among peoples in other West African societies, the mother is very indulgent to her children who as a consequence internalize her norms and imagery and have control of their aggressions. Furthermore, these inhabitants have strong identifications with the family and are held accountable or blamed for their failures so that self-devaluation becomes an integral aspect of the self-system.

The Ghanaian folk ideology interpreted a person's bizarre behavior as a consequence of the influences of witches or of the spirits who have invaded his *kra* or life-force, thereby afflicting his body or his actions. This folk interpretation would seemingly allocate blame for abnormal behavior to forces outside the self; the afflicted person could thus rationalize that his behavior was not his fault. But the very condition of being afflicted by witches or evil spirits was a source of stigma and for which the afflicted person was responsible because of suspected immoral behavior or other unknown deviance.[41, 50] In addition, the man who lost his job or the woman who was barren was socially condemned and blamed. Consequently, the afflicted person would internalize this social blame and become depressed regardless of the rationale for his social failures, because he would be condemned and sometimes socially ostracized. This folk interpretation of external influences upon one's behavior is consistent with psychoanalytic and even sociopsychological versions of depressive reactions. From a psychoanalytic view, the depressed person generally internalizes the hostile person's orientation within his mental system. From a sociopsychological view, the depressed person takes on the job of self-deprecation and sees himself from this reproachful perspective.

In brief, despite the diverse views of the influence of technologically underdeveloped societies and their cultures upon the onset and frequency of manic-depression, it appears that the evidence shows that manic-depressive psychoses, particularly the depressive type, exist with some frequency in these countries but the expressions of and rationale for these disorders varies from those of European prototypes. It means too that these disorders or their absence are not necessarily functions of "racial temperament." Nonetheless, this problem remains one with inconsistent findings and requires further definitive inquiries for conclusive results.

CONCLUSION

In this chapter, I have analyzed some generic and specific issues in psychiatric sociology which affect its theoretical scope, direction, and continuity.

Within the broad field of psychiatric sociology, I have pointed out divergent positions as to its scope. This difference in scope affects the research on the relationship between epidemiological indicators and etiological processes. The interdisciplinary definition of scope encompasses pursuit of genetic, psychogenetic, and other causal factors in addition to the social influences. The sociological view restricts studies to the determination of the etiological relevance of social factors for the different types of disorders; hence, its modes of research are within the competence of a single discipline.

In his research quests, the psychiatric sociologist is limited by conditions outside and inside the discipline. As a nonclinician, he usually lacks direct access to subjects and clinical records; hence, he depends upon the psychiatrist for cooperative inquiry, with the frequent consequence that the topical point of departure is determined by the psychiatrist while the research design is formulated by the sociologist.

Selection of types of research areas, whether by the psychiatrist or the sociologist, affects the continuity of theoretical growth of psychiatric sociology. The problem-centered approach, influenced by community needs, may create discontinuity in theoretical development. By contrast, theory-centered inquiries which aim to fill the gaps of past studies contribute to continuity. But psychiatric sociology is dependent upon the community for subsidizing research; hence it tends to select problems considered urgent by the community, with inevitable discontinuity in theoretical growth.

To illustrate these substantive disagreements, I have focused on research dealing with schizophrenia and manic-depressive psychoses. Data on socioeconomic status, social mobility, and schizophrenia may be interpreted as residual indicators of genetic and/or psychogenetic etiological influences or as indicators of etiological social stresses within the structure of society. Intensive crucial inquiries are required to directly address these competing hypotheses.

In striving for clarity in the relationship between social isolation and schizophrenia, I have argued that social isolation resulting from social rejection seems more malignant than does isolation stemming from clinically accessible contacts. The breadth of this problem and the exploratory findings which have engendered some controversy requires intensive research from several vantage points to derive complete answers.

A representative macrosociological problem is found in the relationship of cultural complexity to schizophrenia and manic-depressive psychoses. Although one position contends that schizophrenia is a disorder predominantly of the complex society, sufficient evidence has demonstrated that it is a universal disorder. This need not indicate that schizophrenia is a product of biopsychological influences but rather points up the occurrence of severe social stress stemming from conflicting social relations in simple societies. Manic-depressive psychosis, especially the depressive type, has likewise been regarded as being characteristic of technologically and culturally advanced peoples. Data on this issue comprise an array of contradictory findings, indicating the need for further cross-cultural analyses.

REFERENCES

1. BEAGLEHOLE, E.: "Cultural Complexity and Psychological Problems." *Psychiatry* 3: 330-352, 1946.
2. BENEDICT, P. K., AND JACKS, I.: "Mental Illness and Primitive Societies." *Psychiatry* 17: 177-189, 1954.
3. CAROTHERS, J. C.: "A Study of Mental Derangement Among Africans and an Attempt to Explain its Peculiarities." *Psychiatry* 11: 47-80, 1948.
4. CLAUSEN, J., AND KOHN, M.: "Social Isolation and Schizophrenia." *American Sociological Review* 20: 265-273, 1955.
5. DEVEREAUX, G.: "A Sociological Theory of Schizophrenia." *Psychoanalytic Review* 26: 315-342, 1939.
6. DOHRENWEND, B. P.: "Social Status and Psychological Disorder: An Issue of Substance and an Issue of Method." *American Sociological Review* 11: 14-34, 1966.
7. DHUNJIBOY, J. E.: "A Brief Resume of the Types of Insanity Commonly Peculiar to the Country." *Journal of Mental Science* 76: 254-255, 1950.
8. DUNHAM, H. W.: *Sociological Theory and Mental Disorders.* Detroit: Wayne State University Press, 1959.
9. DUNHAM, H. W., PHILLIPS, P. AND SRINIVASAN, B.: "A Research Note on Diagnosed Mental Illness and Social Class." *American Sociological Review* 31: 223-227, 1966.
10. FARIS, E.: "Culture Among the Forest Bantu." Pp. 287-288 in *Nature of Human Nature.* New York: McGraw Hill Book Company, 1937.
11. FARIS, R. E. L.: "Cultural Isolation and Schizophrenic Personality." *American Journal of Sociology* 40: 455-456, 1934.
12. FARIS, R. E. L., AND DUNHAM, H. W.: *Mental Disorders in Urban Areas.* Chicago: University of Chicago Press, 1939.
13. FIELD, M.: *Search For Security.* London: Faber and Faber, 1960.
14. GOLDHAMER, H., AND MARSHALL, A.: *Psychoses and Civilization.* New York: Free Press, 1955.
15. GRINKER, R., AND SPIEGEL, J.: *Men Under Stress.* Philadelphia: Blakiston, 1945.
16. JACO, E. G.: "Social Isolation Hypotheses and Schizophrenia." *American Sociological Review* 19: 367-377, 1955.
17. KARDINER, A.: *Psychological Frontiers of Society.* New York: Columbia University Press, 1945.
18. LAPOUSE, R., MONK, M. A., AND TERRIS, M.: "The Drift Hypothesis and Socioeconomic Differentials in Schizophrenia." *American Journal of Public Health* 4:, 978-986, 1956.
19. LEIGHTON, D., AND KLUCKHOHN, C.: *Children of the People.* Cambridge: Harvard University Press, 1948.
20. LEMERT, E.: *Human Deviance: Social Problems and Social Control.* Englewood Cliffs: Prentice-Hall, Inc., 1967.
21. LINDESMITH, A., AND STRAUSS, A.: *Social Psychology.* New York: Holt, Rinehart, and Winston, 1968.
22. LOPATA, H. Z.: "Loneliness: Forms and Components." *Social Problems* 17: 248-262, 1969.
23. LOWENTHAL, M. F.: "Social Isolation and Mental Illness in Old Age." *American Sociological Review* 29: 54-70, 1964.
24. LYSTAD, M. H.: "Social Mobility Among Selected Groups of Schizophrenic Patients." *American Sociological Review* 22: 288-292, 1957.
25. MANIS, J. G., AND B. N. MELTZER (eds.): *Symbolic Interaction.* Boston: Allyn and Bacon, 1967.
26. MORRIS, J.: "Health and Social Class." *Lancet* 1: 303-305, 1959.
27. NEILSON, J. N., AND THOMPSON, G.: *The Engrammes of Psychiatry.* Springfield: Charles C Thomas, 1947.
28. REDLICH, F. C., AND HOLLINGSHEAD, A. B.: "Social Mobility and Mental Illness." *American Journal of Psychiatry* 112: 179-185, 1955.
29. RENNIE, T. A.: "Social Psychiatry: A Definition." *International Journal of Social Psychiatry* 1: 5-13, 1953.
30. ROSE, A. M. (ed.): *Human Behavior and Social Process.* Boston: Houghton Mifflin, and Company, 1962.

31. RUESCH, J.: "Social Psychiatry: An Overview." *Archives of General Psychiatry* 12: 501-509, 1965.
32. SACHS, W.: *Black Hamlet.* Boston: Little Brown and Company, 1947.
33. SCHEFF, T. J.: *Being Mentally Ill.* Chicago: Aldne Publishing Company, 1966.
34. SELIGMAN, C. G.: "Temperament, Conflict and Psychosis in a Stone Age Population." *British Journal of Medical Psychology* 9: 187-202, 1929.
35. SROLE, L., AND ASSOCIATES: *Mental Health in the Metropolis: The Midtown Manhattan Study.* New York: McGraw Hill Book Company, 1962.
36. SROLE, L., AND LANGER, T.: "Social-economic Status Groups: Their Mental Health and Composition." Pp. 33-47 in S. Kirson Weinberg (ed.): *The Sociology of Mental Disorders.* Chicago: Aldine Publishing Company, 1967.
37. TEITZE, C., LEMKAU, P., AND COOPER, M.: "Schizophrenia, Manic-depression and Socioeconomic Status." *American Journal of Sociology* 47: 167-175, 1941.
38. WEINBERG, S. K.: "Combat Neuroses." *American Journal of Sociology* 51: 465-478, 1946.
39. WEINBERG, S. K.: *Society and Personality Disorders.* Englewood Cliffs, N.J.: Prentice-Hall, Inc., 1952.
40. WEINBERG, S. K.: "The Relevance of the Forms of Isolation to Schizophrenia." *International Journal of Social Psychiatry* 13: 33-41, 1956.
41. WEINBERG, S. K.: "Mental Healing and Social Change in West Africa." *Social Problems* 11: 257-269, 1964.
42. WEINBERG, S. K.: "Psychiatric Sociology." Pp. 3-7 in S. Kirson Weinberg (ed.): *The Sociology of Mental Disorders.* Chicago: Aldine Publishing Co., 1967.
43. WEINBERG, S. K.: "Primary Group Therapy, Closest Friendship of the Same Sex: Empirical Analysis," in T. Shibutani (ed.): *Human Nature and Collective Behavior.* New Jersey: Prentice-Hall, 1970, pp. 301-322.
44. WEINBERG, S. K.: *Incest Behavior.* New York: Citadel Press, 1955.
45. DUNHAM, H. W.: "Social Class and Schizophrenia." *American Journal of Orthopsychiatry* 34: 634-642, 1964.
46. LAUBSCHER, B. J. F.: *Custom and Psychopathology.* London: Routledge and Sons, Ltd., 1937.
47. DEMBOWITZ, N., AND CAROTHERS, J. C.: *African Mind on Health and Disease.* Geneva: World Health Organization, 1953.
48. AUBIN, H.: "Introduction A'lude de la Psychribe chez les Noirs." *Annals of Medical Psychologie* 97: 1-29, 1939.
49. TOOTH, G.: *Studies in Mental Illness on the Gold Coast.* London: His Majesty's Press, 1950.
50. WINTROB, R., AND WITKOWER, E. D.: "Witchcraft in Liberia," in Stanley Lesse (ed.): *Psychological Implications: An Evaluation of the Results of Psychotherapy.* Springfield, Illinois: Charles C Thomas, 1968, pp. 1-13.

CHAPTER 3

The Labeling Theory and Mental Illness*

C. RICHARD FLETCHER, PETER K. MANNING, LARRY T. REYNOLDS, AND JAMES O. SMITH

The initial contribution of sociologists to psychiatry came in the form of explications of social factors associated with mental illness. Several studies have shown social factors to be relevant to the etiology, identification, distribution, incidence, and course of mental illness.[9, 6, 23, 25, 15] Other studies have elucidated some of the socially problematic features of diagnosis and prognosis in doctor-patient encounters.[39, 4, 30, 13, 14] In general, the findings of these studies as well as their underlying assumptions were consistent with the established aims and goals of psychiatry. This no doubt contributed to their ready acceptance, together with the fact that psychiatrists had had previous awareness of the relationship between social aspects of health and illness. Examination of the recent history of psychiatry shows that this discipline was welcomed and partially set the stage for contemporary "social psychiatry." Most noteworthy is the fact that the basic assumptions of psychiatry about mental illness, (i.e., that it is a palpable sociopsychological phenomenon, readily identified, isolated, and categorized by medical taxonomies) constituted the framework of inquiry for these sociological studies.

A new perspective on the social implications of mental illness has recently emerged in the process of development. In contrast to the previous reliance on basic psychiatric assumptions, this perspective seriously challenges the traditional medical explanations of mental illness, the applicability of the disease concept to mental illness, and the efficacy and value of psychiatric institutions and treatment techniques. This perspective takes the developmental features

*The authors acknowledge the very helpful comments of Norman Denzin and Horacio Fabrega, Jr. on an earlier draft.

associated with becoming mentally ill and uses them as a framework for analyzing the phenomena of mental illness. Research carried out within this perspective has pointed to the social contingencies which lead to hospitalization, the social effects of hospitalization, and the negative consequences of being treated as mentally ill, whether this occurs in the community prior to medical treatment, during treatment, or in the period that follows treatment. The fact that this counter-perspective has emerged at a time when independent research findings are showing that psychiatric variables, symptomatology, diagnosis, and prognosis, are actually very weak predictors of hospitalization, treatment, and adequate return to the community,[40] has no doubt contributed to the force of its arguments.

In this chapter we critically assess the substance of this theoretical perspective, typically referred to as "labeling theory." We examine the adequacy of the new psychiatric sociology in terms of its concepts, explanations and evidence, and, in a more detailed fashion, evaluate the nature of its challenge to traditional psychiatry. We are specifically concerned with the use of labeling theory in the study of mental disorders, but wish to also consider the overall implications of its use for the sociology of deviance.

Sociologists most identified with the new perspective employ a sociopsychological role theory, drawing on concepts from the theater. In this theory, the self-concept of the deviant, or mentally ill person, is given great importance; it is seen as both a cause and a result of the reactions of specific audiences to the behavior of the actor who plays the role of a deviant. These reactions often lead audiences to assign identities, or labels, to the actor who may then internalize them and allow them to influence his subsequent behavior. Thus, the perspective's basic hypothesis is that the behavior of deviants may be significantly affected by the form of sanctioning they encounter. Messinger and associates[29] summarize this dramaturgical perspective:

> Thus, the dramaturgic analyst conceives the individual as a "performer" whose activities function to create the "appearance" of a "self"—a "character"—for an "audience". . . . Others are related to the individual in terms of their "parts" in putting a "show" together, or witnessing it, of sustaining it, or of disrupting it. . . . The outcome of interest to the analyst is the "effective" creating of a "character" which, by "taking in" the "audience" or failing to do so, will permit the individual to continue a rewarding line of activity or to avoid an unrewarding one, or which will result in his being "discredited." Finally, the dramaturgic analyst seems to make mental patients of us all, for he conceives the individual as "staging" *fundamental* qualities: aspects of self taken for granted with *intimate* others [p. 104].

This dramaturgical perspective uses the concept of career that is consistent with role theory and which minimizes the emphasis on individual characteristics which is prominent in traditional psychiatry. The explanatory power derived from the use of the career concept is one of the primary contributions of this new perspective. The behavior of individuals who subsequently become mental patients is viewed within progressive stages of a natural social history which neglects " . . . unique outcome . . . in favor of such changes over time as are basic and common to the members of a social category"[19] [p. 127]. Internal characteristics such as self-identity, are linked with external ones such as role, office, or position. The concept of career entails a set of steps within a structure, or system, and includes an individual's perception and definition of the social situation. The concept thus lends itself nicely to the explication that there are linkages that exist between external and internal characteristics at specified stages.

We employ the career concept to organize our subsequent discussion. Our critical focus is primarily on the work of Goffman and Scheff. We consider the following stages in the "career of the mental patient": prelabeling, labeling, inpatient status, and return to the community.

FIRST CAREER STAGE: PRELABELING

In the earliest stages of a mental patient's career, some behavior is manifested which warrants the identification of mental illness. This is explicated by Scheff,[37] who has made an important attempt to synthesize sociological thought regarding the role of the mentally ill. He presents a theoretical model in which the behavior of the "sick" actor is conceptualized as residual deviance. His concept in turn hinges upon a notion of residual rules:

Most norm violations do not cause the violator to be labeled as mentally ill, but as ill-mannered, ignorant, sinful, criminal, or perhaps just harried, depending on the type of norm involved. (Or potential definers may deny that the deviance even warrants labeling). After exhausting these categories . . . there is always a residue of the most diverse kinds of violations for which the culture provides no explicit label. These are unnameable and unthinkable forms of deviance . . . For convenience these violations are lumped together into a residual category: witchcraft, spirit possession, or, in our own society, mental illness [pp. 31-34].

Scheff[37] suggests the following examples of "residual rules," which we have arranged in order of severity [pp. 32, 36, 38]:

1. When engaged in conversation, face your partner, rather than look directly away from him.

2. When gazing toward a conversational partner, look toward his eyes, rather than, say, toward his forehead.

3. Stand at a proper conversational distance, neither one inch away nor across the room.

4. Do not indulge in an "away" in a socially unacceptable context. (Scheff accepts Goffman's[20] coinage of an "away" to refer to those "inward emigrations from the gathering, coming under the psychiatric rubric of withdrawal.")

45

5. Do not exhibit such "psychiatric symptoms as withdrawal, hallucinations, continual muttering, posturing, etc."

We take issue with Scheff[37] when he characterizes these examples and "norms over which consensus is so complete that the members of the group appear to take them for granted, thus being *neither verbalized nor explicitly taught*" [p. 32]. We suggest that for each of these examples there are verbalized and explicitly taught exhortations such as (1 and 2) "Look me in the eye and say that"; (3) "Don't crowd me," or "Stand up to him like a man"; (4) "Where have *you* been?" or "Join the party"; (5) "You're out of your tree!" or even "You should see a psychiatrist," all of which can come into play when this rule-breaking behavior occurs.

We would suggest that Scheff's concept of residual deviance should not replace the earlier, but similar concept of Garfinkel[17] called "constitutive rules of social interaction." As defined by Garfinkel, these rules are not so much specifications of substantive behavior as they are criteria of the possible locale, numbers of participants, and order of action an individual assumes must be chosen by himself and others in social interaction. These most nearly resemble ground rules or basic rules of a game. They are largely implicit in that one is not aware of them until one has broken them, but the breaking of them does not necessarily warrant one being thrust into a category of deviance. Thus, in contrast to Scheff's analysis, the crucial deviance that occurs during the prelabeling phase may be the breaking of basic rules of social interaction rather than the residual rules.

SECOND CAREER STAGE: LABELING AND/OR PSYCHIATRIC REFERRAL

An assumption held by most labeling theorists is that the designation "mentally ill" is so unquestionably pernicious that it should be abolished. Failing in this, it is subtly advocated that the designation should be circumvented by patients who are clever enough to in the treatment institution. Presumably such patients might adopt the style of the character Randall McMurphy in *One Flew Over the Cuckoo's Nest* who survived brutal custodial hospitalization for a time by stubbornly refusing to internalize the mental illness label.

Labeling theorists do not clearly formulate the transition from a socially defined status of normal to one of mental illness. Looking first at the dynamics of the small primary groups in which instrumental or expressive failure is first likely to become apparent, research by Sampson and associates[35] and Yarrow and coworkers[43] shows most families possess a great capacity to force a disturbed member into an accommodative relationship, keeping him within the family unit in spite of severe difficulties. Eventually, persons around the patient not only perceive his deviant behavior, but strongly hold the view that he had been a mentally disturbed person for some time. This does not necessarily relate to a particular quality of behavior, but only refers to the point at which the audience begins to interpret his behavior as being that of a mentally ill person needing help. As Goffman says, the "axial event" may be an occurrence within the social system surrounding the patient rather than within the patient himself. One example of this was observed by one of the authors at the admission hearings of a Midwestern state mental hospital: a family was able to tolerate the bizarre behavior of a daughter until they planned to have a wedding party at their home, at which point they arranged to have her permanently hospitalized. Lemert[26] provided an earlier example:

> Commitment may be a sign of changed tolerance for the deviant rather than of an exaggeration of his psychotic behavior . . . . even such a simple thing as overtaxing the laundry facilities of a growing family by incontinent elders may be the social break leading to hospitalization. In a sociological time-analysis of the phenomena of institutionalization it is clear that the tolerance quotient must be related to such things as family life cycles [p. 373].

Outside the immediate family and friendship circles, where relationships are more public, formalized, and tenuous, there are fewer long-term opportunities for negotiating such an accommodation; likewise there are fewer losses to the offended groups if they fail to do so. Goffman[19] would classify these considerations as "career contingencies":

> Separating those offenses which could have been used as grounds for hospitalizing the offender from those that are so used, one finds a vast number of what students of occupation call career contingencies. Some of these contingencies in the mental patient's career have been suggested, if not explored, such as socio-economic status, visibility of the offense, proximity to mental hospital, amount of treatment and facilities available, community regard for the type of treatment given and available hospitals, and so on. . . . the societies' official view is that inmates of mental hospitals are there primarily because they are suffering from mental illness. However, in the degree that the 'mentally ill' outside hospitals numerically approach or surpass those inside hospitals, one could say that mental patients distinctively suffer not from mental illness, but from contingencies [pp. 134, 135].

Evident in this statement is a focus upon the control and exploitation of the actor by those around him as he moves from familial to public exposure, victimization and mortification, within a "funnel of betrayal," as Goffman[19] describes it.

The centrality of the labeling event in labeling theory is evidenced by Scheff's[37] hypothesis that, "Among residual deviants, labeling is the single most important cause of careers of residual deviance" [p. 92]. Working toward a definition of labeling, he states:

> The societal reaction to rule-breaking (although usually denial) is not always denial, however. In a small proportion of cases the reaction goes the other

way, *exaggerating* and at the same time distorting the extent and degree of the violation. This pattern of exaggeration . . . we call 'labeling' . . . When labeling first occurs, it merely *gives a name* to rule-breaking . . . (But) It may create a social type, a pattern of *'symptomatic' behavior* in conformity with the stereotyped expectations of others[37] [pp. 81, 92].

However, as with Scheff's definition of residual deviance, his definition of labeling is difficult to operationalize. How is the "exaggeration" to be identified by the researcher?

One suggestion here is by the *name given* to the rule-breaking. But to focus on naming presents two difficulties: First, it would seem logically impossible to give a name to a form of behavior defined as "unnameable and unthinkable," as Scheff's definition of residual deviance indicates.

Second, if giving a name is an essential element of labeling, then we question whether labeling does in fact occur for numerous aggressive and sociopathic deviants who become mental patients without their interpersonal community necessarily applying the term "mentally ill." It is highly questionable whether the designation of mental illness is applied with widespread consensus to deviants who continue to uphold their own behavior as being proper while derogating the dominant norms as illegitimate, especially in the cases of acting-out patients who undergo hospitalization without resocialization. This deviant category has been referred to as "enemy deviance"[22] and as "political deviance."[24, 33]

Even families of psychotic patients persist in normalizing the condition; for example, they define the strange behavior in purely organic terms (e.g., "a case of nerves") which have been understandably caused (e.g., by "overwork"). Being under psychiatric care is not the precise equivalent of being labeled mentally ill. This is a point requiring more clarification in current labeling theory.

Scheff[38] has indicated elsewhere that he is not committed to the designation, *per se*. He cites Phillips' study of "reaction to psychiatric symptoms under conditions where a psychiatric label had, and had not, been applied." Scheff[38] continues, "This study demonstrates very convincingly the effects of 'denial' and 'labeling' on the 'recognition' of mental illness" [p. 22]. Since the Phillips study did not deal with the label of mental illness *per se*, but rather with the seeking of psychiatric help, we can only assume that Scheff is content in this instance to ignore the concept of mental illness as an unnecessary aspect of the labeling process.

Another indication of Scheff's[37] view that the designation mental illness is nonessential to the labeling process is found in his citation of Glass' observation that military neuropsychiatric casualities may not become mentally ill if they are kept with their unit, but many become chronically impaired when removed from the unit to a hospital. Scheff then comments, "That is, their deviance is stabilized by the labelling process, which is implicit in their removal and hospitalization" [p. 83]. If the label can be implicit, then at least it could be said that the research utility of the concept is brought into serious question. At most, Scheff is self-contradictory.

A second clue as to how one identifies the exaggeration of the degree of norm violation is suggested in Scheff's[37] definition of labeling. The deviant is presumably expected to conform to a *stereotype* of mental illness:

> The stereotype of insanity is "learned in early childhood" and is "continually reaffirmed" so that a deviant "accepts this preferred role as the only available framework within which he can organize his behavior" [p. 84].

If such a stereotypical role does in fact exist, we would expect the behavior of the mentally ill to match it with some precision. But we believe it does not. We question Scheff's suggestion that there is a substantial correspondence between a cultural stereotype of "madness" or "insanity" and actual mental illness behavior, particularly in cases of sociopathy and chronic schizophrenia. This suggests that Scheff has either underestimated the complexities of the stereotype or overestimated the priority of the cultural stereotype as the role model for the residual deviant. In sum, the concept of the stereotype is not a sufficient clue as to when and under what circumstances the deviant actor commits himself to the role of being mentally ill.

Scheff also argues that labeling tends to stabilize the deviance and then builds this conclusion on a series of propositions which each have a place in producing the final result of mental illness. The movement from normality to mental illness parallels Lemert's[27] distinction between primary and secondary deviance:

> Primary deviation, as contrasted with secondary deviation is perceived as normal variation—a problem of everyday life . . . dealt with reciprocally in the context of established status relationships . . . and has only marginal implications for the status and psychic structure of the person concerned.
>
> Secondary deviation refers to the individual's responses to the moral problems of stigmatization, punishments, segregation and social control, created by the societal reaction to his deviance. Their problems generate for him a specialized organization of social roles, identity and self-regarding attitudes to the extent that his life is organized around the facts of deviance [pp. 40, 41].

Some specific elements of the label mental illness presumably operate to stabilize the deviance. These are its connotations that the deviant's condition is pervasive of his entire character structure, that it is chronic, and that the condition disqualifies him as a responsible member of society. We consider these in turn:

Pervasiveness. Scheff, Goffman, and Lemert do not discuss those instances in which the deviant might find, on assuming the mentally ill role, that within the concept of illness there exist diagnoses which are *not* pervasive, but instead are compartmentalized or peripheral to an essentially normal organism. For example, the nonglobal concept of the "allergy to alcohol" has been used with some success by Alcoholics Anonymous; further exploration of the relevance of such a concept for certain forms of psychological disorder may be fruitful.

Chronicity. These writers imply that the diagnosis of mental illness carries an implication of incurability or permanence. It may be that acute, transitory disorders serve as more accurate analogies for the course of most mental disorders.

Nonresponsibility. Labelling theorists have argued that the mental patient is cut off from the normative system of reward and punishment because he is not considered accountable as the causal agent of his actions.[10] This is due to the alleged connotations of the diseased model of disordered behavior. Within the diagnostic subculture, the patient's communications are not taken at face value; they are reinterpreted, or discounted as manifestations of underlying symptoms of the illness. He is supposedly left hanging in moral space, disqualified as a social actor.

Assuming the mentally ill person is not held accountable for his problem would actually tend to *lessen* the stigma of the mental illness label. If we accept Garfinkel's[45] conceptualization, no degradation ceremony is complete if the noxious causal agent is located outside the deviant individual. However, this exemption from accountability is not a general rule. Laymen still mistrust psychiatry's efforts to limit laymen's right to make moral judgments. Indeed, as Zubin[44] puts it, "the persistence of the 'stigma' that clings to mental illness is perhaps at least in part to be explained by the man in the street's resistance to any determinist encroachment on his personal responsibility." Fletcher[11] found empirical evidence of this persistent moralism. Fifty working-class couples and fifty middle-class couples were presented with fictitious case descriptions of an aggressive and withdrawn person, and asked to assess: (1) the extent of *deviance* in terms of unusualness and incompatibility; (2) the extent of the described actor's *responsibility* for his own behavior, in terms of whether he caused his own behavior (accountability) and could amend it himself (amendability); and (3) whether the respondent would *refer* these cases to a psychiatrist.

The respondents' estimates of deviance were *not* found to be highly correlated with their prediction toward psychiatric referral. Analysis of the responsibility variable resulted in a pattern which was theoretically understandable. High assignments of accountability were found to make positive contributions to respondents' referral decisions. For middle-class respondents, the high estimate of accountability strengthened the unusualness-referral relationship, while for the working-class respondents, the high estimate of accountability strengthened the *incompatibility*-referral relationship. It appears that the general public, although perhaps giving lip-service to psychiatric orientations, act as if they have defined some forms of mental illness, particularly the aggressive and sociopathological forms, as being morally wrong rather than an indication of sickness. They may expect the psychiatrist to behave, therefore, as a moralist rather than as a physician who must reflect neutral values.

THIRD CAREER STAGE: INPATIENT
ADMISSION, TREATMENT, AND DISCHARGE

The central work on the impatient phase of the career is Goffman's *Asylums*.[19] Goffman describes the processes of the inpatient phase within the confines of the total institution:

A total instition may be defined as a place of residence and work where a large number of like-situated individuals, cut off from the wider society for an appreciable period of time, together lead an enclosed, formally administered round of life. Prisons serve as a clear example, providing we appreciate that what is prison-like about prisons is found in institutions whose members have broken no laws [p. x].

Goffman's work is characterized by a commitment to the subjective experience of the patient and a sentimental attachment to the underdog; these features are at one and the same time the strength and weakness of his work.

The main focus is on the world of the inmate, not the world of the staff. A chief concern is to develop a sociological version of the structure of the self [p. x].

We now focus on several difficulties that appear in Goffman's treatment of the inpatient phase.

Unclear scope and intent of the total institution concept

In his conceptualization of the total institution, Goffman attempts to draw together the bureaucratic nature and the communal or strongly controlled nature of the institution. Levinson and Gallagher[28] summarize his intent:

Goffman's work represents the first large scale effort to examine the mental hospital from the view point of its patient members and to relate their situation to those of inmates in other highly segregated autocratically structured institutions. He concerns himself with the features of institutional practice in everyday interaction common to those various settings. Supplementing his own immediate observations with judicious selections from the writing of articulate ex-inmates . . ., he achieves a fresh and critical perspective—'worm's eye view', as it were. The total institution is seen as a specialized instrumentality in the service of man's inhumanity to man. Goffman describes and classifies the myriad form of betrayal, mortification, soul stripping, and identity transformation to which inmates are subjected. All of this is justified, in each locale, by the currently favored ideology psychiatry, military, penal, religious, or political [p. 19].

Levinson and Gallagher proceed to point out ambiguity in Goffman's work. For example, not all mental hospitals are total institutions. Moreover, it is not clear whether Goffman intends this work to be a case study of a single institution, a representative case study generalizable to all total institutions, a case study of a mental hospital which is a total institution, or a compendium of all the important dimensions of total institutions no matter what their goals, values, social structures, or clientele. But Levinson and Gallagher may be taking Goffman too literally. Goffman suggests almost a metaphoric usage of the concept of the total institution throughout *Asylums*. For example, he notes that

> . . . none of the elements I will describe seems peculiar to total institutions, and none seems to be shared by every one of them; what is distinctive about total institutions is that each exhibits to an intense degree many items in this family of attributes [p. 5].

Thus, the concept of the total institution is one of his many fictive devices for examining the range of human behavior; his investment in the terms and associated concepts, however, seems inadequate.

Goffman fails to provide indications of the transitions that occur from one stage to the next in the patient career. The point at which the inpatient phase begins may be the point at which the patient subjectively identifies himself as being mentally ill, or it may be the point at which formal agencies of social control designate him to be so, or it may occur simply with the entrance into an institution.

Model of Bureaucracy

Another point of criticism which may be levelled at Goffman's concept of the total institution is that he fails to be explicit in his commitment to the bureaucratic model and all that such a model entails. His polarized, two-party "worlds"—staff and patient—seem to hang in organizational space. There is no reference to the disparate *social positions* of staff and patient as a primary determinant of their different role behavior, views of illness, efficiency, and devotion to curing or caring. Goffman acknowledges that the mental hospital as a total institution is essentially bureaucratic in nature, but he goes little beyond this. For example, he notes that:

> The handling of many human needs by the bureaucratic organization of whole blocks of people—whether or not this is a necessary or effective means of social organization in the circumstances—is the key fact of total institutions. From this follow certain important implications [p. 6].

What are the "important implications" of the bureaucracy of which Goffman speaks? He says, "The staff-inmate split is one major implication of the bureaucratic management of large blocks of persons." This means that (1) a small staff whose chief activity is surveillance can supervise the patients; (2) each grouping tends to view the other in terms of a hostile, antagnostic stereotype; (3) social mobility between the two strata, by definition, is virtually nonexistent; and (4) the staff controls communication from inmates to higher levels of staff. Goffman indicates a second major implication of the bureaucratization of the mental hospital: work. We learn that work takes on a different meaning in the inmate culture than in the outside world.

Certainly Goffman's abbreviated treatment of the bureaucratic nature of total institutions and its implications represent an over-simplification. His work is replete with illustrations of the dehumanizing and oppressive features of such institutions. We suggest that these features are embedded in the bureaucratic nature of the total institution. Goffman helpfully catalogues the types of human relationships and behaviors that occur throughout bureaucracies in our society, albeit in extreme cases. Bureaucracy is a structure of human relations based upon hierarchical alignment and dominance, with each higher status exercising dominance over those below. In the mental hospital, the patient has the lowest position in the hierarchy. In Goffman's type of polarization, the patient is dominated by the total system, having few or no rights or privileges of office, let alone duties or power. Although Goffman is concerned with the total institution as a context of the self, he scarcely acknowledges that by determining the position of the individual within the organization, it is the bureaucratic structure which determines his roles and social self.

Goffman views the organization as being static. His organization lacks a dynamic that would allow for or bring about change. While the organization has the power to transform selves, it is apparently unaffected by those persons who constitute its human fabric. The patient self is alleged to undergo radical changes, but not so for the staff self. Goffman[19] sees the "secondary adjustments" of patients, the ways they utilize unauthorized ends or means in the organization to "get around the organization's assumptions about what he should do and as a consequence be," primarily as "contained" within the organization [p. 189]. These secondary adjustments are the means by which the patients carve out an autonomy of the self, which would otherwise be denied by the organization. Although these flavor the system, give it life and humor, and restore the innovative autonomy which is characteristic of men, they do not fundamentally alter the organization. Presumably, this would occur if disruptive secondary adjustments were to prevail. Interestingly enough, although he mentions the existence of "disruptive secondary adjustments," he does not deal with them in *Asylums*.

Goffman's view of the structure of the mental hospital is in contrast to that of Strauss and associates[42] who made a study of several Chicago mental hospitals. They argue that the psychiatric hospital is a dynamic, almost fluid set of relationships existing among professional and organizational segments, loosely bound together only by a vague concept of improving the state of the patient's health. In this case, the patient's fate is far from being regarded as structurally ordained; it is rather a function of negotiation and bargaining by organizational and professional-ideological segments within the hospital. This view contrasts Goffman's apparent commitment to a rather determinant, monolithic view of the structure of the mental hospital in which there is a property of implacability about the organization; a lack of dynamics or resiliency. This approach consequently does not provide for incidental events which might affect the patient, or for meaningful intervention by a higher authority.

Goffman does not take into consideration the impact of technology—for example, the development of tranquilizers, upon the treatment process and hospital organization. This may well be a function of the time at which the study was undertaken since he does mention shock therapy and its use. As Perrow[32] has pointed out, the role of psychiatric technology is important in the dynamics of mental hospital organization. In particular, he argues that drugs have been singularly crucial in the modification of mental hospitals into more therapeutically oriented environments. Perrow, however, goes to the opposite extreme from Goffman and suggests that social alteration or reforms in an organizational sense are relatively unimportant, if not impossible, without technological change.

Patient Culture

Goffman's oversimplification of the organizational structure of the mental hospital resembles his attitude towards the treatment of the patient culture. With Caudill,[5] he views the patient as always being acted upon, but never being able to act effectively on the organization. Goffman's patient[19] is able to erect a strong informal organization and create cliques, occasionally transforming rules and staff intentions to his own use, but presumably has little impact upon the bureaucratic organization or formal structure of the hospital. Both Goffman's and Scheff's conception of the self-as-object resembles quite closely a structurally deterministic or over-socialized conception of the self.

In contrast, Roth,[34] Strauss and associates,[42] and Levinson and Gallagher[28] see the patient as being a potential source of power in the hospital with valid claims, demands to be met, resources to be utilized, and the impact to encourage change. These writers argue that the larger the long-term population in the institution, the greater the potential influence of the inmate body. At the risk of assuming equivalence between mental patients and other types of patients, Roth's insightful treatment of the tuberculosis patient should be cited. He documents these patients' power and ingenuity in influencing doctors, seeking and gaining information, avoiding rules, and pressuring physicians for decisions. Seemingly, such a patient culture would generate a modicum of power with which they could act upon the structure of the situation and hence alter their own fates.

In Goffman's patient world, however, this does not occur. Perhaps he is correct in his analysis, although he does not develop a theoretical explanation for it. Had Goffman taken into account the essential features of bureaucracy, i.e., dominance, coercion, and the hierarchical alignment of power relationships throughout the organization, he could have accounted for the fact that even in the face of the patient culture, the essentials of the power structure are not altered; the staff still dominates the patients. This may be even more pronounced in short-term treatment situations marked by relatively acute conditions, brief periods of hospitalization, and little personal contact with physicians.

Mental patients, along with prisoners, students, and professors have latent identities which become the basis for differentiated subcultures, role types, and transitory cliques. There is some evidence to suggest[46] that these latent identities, particularly those involving compatible socialization to fill the patient role in the doctor-patient relationship, lead to more favorable treatment outcomes. Thus, treatment in Goffman's total institution takes on the ironic character of the dilemma faced by Joseph Heller's hero in the black comedy *Catch 22*. If the patient wishes to "get well" he must publicly admit to illness, shake off old identities, and the stability associated with these role performances and begin to react to himself and others as a mental patient should; that is, as one does who needs help. This shaking off of old identities, Goffman emphasizes, shatters the stability of the patient's interpersonal ties and leads to his inability to perform actions which suggest normality. Hence, as Erikson has argued, the very process of "treatment" creates the deviance it is intended to rehabilitate. ". . . (the patient) is left in the exposed situation of one who has to *look* incompetent even while learning to become the exact opposite."

This is a prime example of the dramaturgical analysis of conflicting role demands, providing a case for a general critique. Messinger and coworkers[29] assert that there are important distinctions between the analyst's and the actor's perspectives on performances. They summarize the difficulties which, when undetected, may lead many readers to assume that all action in a system *is* an ongoing drama:

> The analyst and his readers run the risk of considering the dramaturgic framework to represent his subjects' model of the world. Because 'impression management' is critical in the analyst's scheme of things, because in any situation it is this dimension that he attends to, he may leave the impression that this is the way things 'are' as his subjects see things—or at least that, if they could be brought to be honest for a bit, they would see and admit that this is the case. There is, of course, no justification for this . . . The dramaturgic analyst does not claim that the actor is aware of the impressive functions of his activities . . . But, although in the dramaturgic vision the actor does not attend to the impressive effects of his activities as impressive effects, he nonetheless exhibits a remarkable ability to produce the right effect at just the right time, or, short of this, to correct for the errors he and his teammates may make. How is this accomplished? . . . Is the actor merely the outcome of a dynamicized set of 'organizational principles' which shove and haul him about without his awareness? . . . Anyone committed to an understanding of everyday life and of the 'actor's world' must cope with such questions, . . .

Finally, the theatrical simile may encourage the analyst to forget another important aspect of any everyday actor's communications: the actor is communicating about himself, and this constrains the attitude he may take toward the qualities he projects . . .

He does not, finally, experience life as theater. He does not expect the curtain to ring down, returning what came before to the realm of make-believe. He is constrained to be what he claims, and mental patients suggest that these constraints operate 'inside' the individual as well as 'on' him. Indeed, his need to believe in himself seems even stronger than his need to be certain that others entertain a particular view of him. The basic task joined by mental patients would seem to be the locating and fixing of the reality of themselves. In this, they differ from stage actors; who cannot remain 'on' with impunity. And in this, mental patients represent us all [pp. 108, 109].

The release process has received little attention from labeling theory perhaps because discharge itself suggests there may be some patients who benefit from treatment. Scheff,[37] in considering data on release contingencies, suggests that the type of hospital to which the patient was committed, the patient's age, and length of confinement influence release rates. Older, long confinement patients in receiving hospitals are less likely to be released even if they have little or slight impairment. He argues that these patients are perhaps most dependent upon relatives to support their release because they may be wards of the state. The earlier findings of Hollingshead and Redlich[23] on the impact of class on prognosis, type of therapy and its effectiveness, would suggest that a further bias exists in release rates. These studies underscore the social and miminize the psychiatric factors affecting release. Scheff estimates that approximately 43 per cent of the patients in mental hospitals remain there for nonpsychiatric reasons.

These and other observations we have surveyed echo a familiar sociological theme: institutions do not so much solve the problems with which they deal as they manage the shape and form of them, and in diverse ways reinforce their continued existence. To conceive of mental hospitals as being *solely* a locus of cures for mental illness is now totally discredited. The new social psychiatry, as Scheff explicitly notes, focuses on people who have been adjudged or labelled mentally ill under the medical assumptions that untreated illness is potentially more dangerous than are attempts at intervention and that all illness has an unalterable downward course. There is little attention paid to several other possible types of persons:

1. Those who resist all attempts at character modification; that is, those patients who physically pass through the stages of the model, but do not identify themselves as mentally ill, nor suffer any serious consequences from the experience. There may be resources (for example, psychological, familial) which insulate the person from negative reactions and imputation of deviance.

56

2. Those who benefit from treatment, such as the acutely disturbed person, and return to the community. The success of some types of organic treatments such as electroconvulsive therapy and drugs may provide the patient with the interpretation that his illness is transitory rather than chronic and recurring. Little consideration is given to the conditions under which the label endures or when it fails to endure.

Several studies have dealt with the relative power of sociological and psychiatric variables in predicting rates of rehospitalization,[1, 15, 31] the impact of the stigma of a mentally ill relative on family relationships and attitudes,[40] and familial accommodation to the ex-patient as well as his accommodation to the family.[36] While no resolution of the relative predictive power of the two sets of variables was achieved in these studies, they do tend to offer a more balanced perspective: social factors show low correlations with rehospitalization, and psychiatric factors appear to intervene between social characteristics and types of outcome.

Goffman[20] has devoted a long essay to the general subject of stigma; the signs of moral inferiority which are potentially discrediting to a person. He has also been concerned with the conditions under which stigma can become virtually discrediting. This constitutes a significant issue for concern. It has been asserted that there is a generally unfavorable conception of mental illness in American society; ex-mental patients, unlike ex-socialites, or ex-football players, are potentially discreditable. If "discovered," this identity may result in a hostile or rejecting reaction, particularly from those with whom previous interactional ties had been disrupted, violated, or bruised by inappropriate behavior with people standing in relationships of an enduring, intimate, and constraining nature, that is, family, friends, and neighbors. But Goffman does not focus on these phenomena, directing his attention instead toward the violation of rules of etiquette governing people in less intimate relationships.

Stigma appears to be a fairly pervasive fact in the lives of a considerable number of mental patients. Spitzer and Denzin[40] summarize the differential impact as follows:

> Stigma or sensitivity regarding psychiatric hospitalization of a household member was found to be associated with the degree of inappropriate behavior of the patient after he returned home. Stigma was also associated with the social class of the family as well as with certain personality traits of family members. Sensitivity to stigma was most pronounced within upper class families and among family members characterized by feelings of isolation, frustration and withdrawal . . . Cumming and Cumming show that feelings of stigma are not equally distributed among various segments of two psychiatric populations. In general, high stigma was concentrated within the less severe diagnostic categories such as neurosis, among females not well integrated into family networks, among well-integrated females who had a

leadership role within the family, and among the most recently discharged patients [pp. 385, 386].

With regard to posthospital adjustment of patients to their families, Freeman and Simmons[15] found that higher expectations of performance, such as returning to normal tasks around the house, coupled with a lower tolerance of deviance led to higher rates of rehospitalization for middle class female patients. The same factors appear to account for greater incidence of rehospitalization from conjugal as opposed to parental families.[40]

SUMMARY

The current interest in the field of psychiatric sociology is at least in part a result of the work of three sociologists: Erving Goffman, Thomas Scheff, and to a lesser extent, Edwin Lemert. The thematic similarity in their conceptual foci and their methodological inclinations are central to the currently dominant orientation in the field. These writers are dramatistic interactionists, and we have noted the ways in which this metaphoric stance is difficult to evaluate with respect to the nature of the relationship that exists between actor and observer. Likewise we have pointed to the often fictive nature of the concepts, and the exaggeration the perspective lends to some facets of the behavior of the mentally ill. Above all, the perspective is a sociopsychological role theory which deals best with relationships between the self and social setting. A price is paid for the focus upon interaction: many psychiatric variables and etiological explanations are minimized and complex social structures, for example, bureaucracies are sometimes grossly simplified. For example, there is no evidence that psychiatric variables do not account for a considerable variation in admission, treatment, prognosis, and rehospitalization. The contribution of psychiatric sociology is precisely that it challenges the psychiatric explanation and reinvigorates sociological explanations with a fresh and important line of argument; a totally one-sided approach sharply reduces the potential of this contribution.

In these analyses, the patient is seen as a passive object, locked into a total institution; he has little capacity to alter his fate and possesses ingenuity only in his obsequious accommodations to rigid demands. There is little attempt to clarify the extent to which the patient can modify this environment. With the emphasis upon exploitation and the ongoing debunking of psychiatry which are characteristic of this stance, little attention is given to the possible positive functions of patienthood. For example, electroconvulsive or drug therapy may provide a successful treatment for some patients. Many ironies are captured by our writers, but the one they fail to discuss is the "successful mental patient."

There are basic methodological weaknesses in the material we have considered. In spite of brilliance in observation and ingenuity in research tactics, the dramaturgists fail to define precisely many of their most central concepts such as residual deviance, career, primary and secondary deviation, total institution, and labeling. We have suggested that researchable definitions of these concepts seem difficult to construct. For example, referral behavior seems more essential than naming in Scheff and Goffman's versions of the labeling process. For this reason, we suggest that the central concept should designate referral behavior rather than naming behavior. It is misleading to imply that the essential and sufficient process in the societal endorsement of the mentally ill role is attaching the label of mental illness to the deviant; the more crucial event may be that the individual is referred for outside help, irrespective of the particular label of mental illness. Thus, the concept of labeling without clarification seems insufficiently precise as well as insufficiently comprehensive.

Likewise, there are operational reasons for bypassing the term mental illness. When an interviewer mentions the term mental illness to a lay respondent, the normative response is an acquiescent and stereotypical overlay of verbalization which is tenuously related (if at all) to his actual behavioral response towards the deviant. The more fruitful research stategy should therefore be not simply to delineate the public's definitions and attitudes surrounding the label mental illness but rather to discover behavior responses to specific forms of deviant behavior. It is then possible to approach the central issue of whether this reponse would include the referral of the deviant for help outside of his immediate interpersonal network.[10]

If case descriptions of deviant behavior are utilized as stimuli during an interview in this effort, care should be taken to justify the nature and severity of each attribute of the case in terms of the aims of the study. Fletcher's cases, for example, isolated the variable of the vector of social interaction, namely aggressive behavior in contrast to withdrawn behavior. Extending the work of several previous researchers including Star[41] and Bergen,[3] he controlled other elements in the case descriptions so that the symptoms of both cases were: (1) sudden in onset, (2) of six months duration, (3) occurring frequently and globally i.e., "no matter where he is," (4) paranoid in ideation and affect, (5) subacute rather than dramatically florid.

Future researchers would hopefully continue to isolate variables in this manner, by constructing the required number of pairs of case descriptions with each pair being contrasted in terms of a single variable.

Gibbs[18] raises an important problem by pointing out that dramaturgic theorists are unclear on whether they are attempting to explain the deviant behavior itself or the response of others to a particular form of deviant behavior. Gove[21] asks a similar question in a recent attempt to adduce the limited empirical evidence on the question of the societal reaction theory of mental illness. According to Gove, the research indicates that in the processes of labeling, hospitalization, and posthospital rehabilitation, the performance of the individual is more important than the societal expectations of his performance or the social reactions to his deviant behavior. He, like Gibbs, is attempting to redress the balance between individual and social forces in the theoretical understanding of mental illness.

59

Although the natural history-career approach has been employed by the dramaturgists, the points at which transition occurs from one phase of the career to the next are unclear. Although Scheff and Goffman have both done ingenious research, they have only begun to chart points of transition in broad outlines. An example is the issue of whether labeling is *sufficient* cause for launching a deviant career. Perhaps it is fruitful, as Scheff suggests, to examine a set of factors in the context of a naturalistic model of causation which addresses the social construction of moral meanings as a process, or series of steps, each with its own cause or causes, with no single event setting off a domino-like chain.[2,7]

A final mention should be made of the importance of the norms violated in the deviance called mental illness. The nature of the norms violated at different career stages seem to be quite different. Scheff places emphasis on "residual rules," a concept derived from Goffman's analysis of encounters. These are most relevant to matters of self-respect or deference among strangers, and may not be crucial in distinctions between inappropriate and appropriate behavior among intimates. The ways in which the family group defines illness may require detailed case studies, such as those of Messinger and his associates.[29] We need further study of the time-ordered formulation of a definition of mental illness central to the first two career stages; likewise, further exploration of the definition of recovery is needed. This suggests further that quite different things are being explained at each level, and that the global concept of mental illness must be viewed in light of *situational specification*. This in turn calls for a natural history which includes emphasis upon a different set of variables and concepts at each stage. We would thus continue to deal with the properties of events and social categories as they are modified and transformed in the process of movement through the career stages, and continue the revision of conceptions of mental illness begun so significantly by Goffman, Scheff, and others.

REFERENCES

1. ANGRIST, S. A., et al.: *Women After Treatment.* New York: Appleton-Century-Crofts, 1968.
2. BECKER, H. S.: *The Outsiders,* New York: Free Press, 1963.
3. BERGEN, B. J.: Social Class, Symptoms and Mental Illness. Unpublished Ph. D. dissertation. Harvard University, 1962.
4. BLOOM, S.: *The Doctor and His Patient.* New York: Free Press, 1963.
5. CAUDILL, W.: *The Psychiatric Hospital as a Small Society.* Cambridge: Harvard University Press, 1958.
6. CLAUSEN, J., AND KOHN, M.: "The Ecological Approach to Social Psychiatry." *American Journal of Sociology* 60: 140-151, 1954.
7. DOUGLAS, J. D.: *The Social Meanings of Suicide.* Princeton: Princeton University Press, 1967.
8. ERIKSON, K. T.: "Patient Role and Social Uncertainty: A Dilemma of the Mentally Ill." *Psychiatry* 20: 263-674, 1957.
9. FARIS, R. E. L., AND DUNHAM, H.: *Mental Disorders in Urban Areas.* Chicago: University of Chicago Press, 1939.
10. FLETCHER, C. R.: "Attributing Responsibility to the Deviant: A Factor in Psychiatric Referrals by the General Public." *Journal of Health and Social Behavior* 8: 185-196, 1967.
11. FLETCHER, C. R.: "Social Class Variations in Psychiatric Referral of Withdrawn and Aggressive Case Descriptions." *Social Problems* 16: 227-242, 1968.

12. FLETCHER, C. R.: "Measuring Community Mental Health Attitudes by Means of Hypothetical Case Descriptions." *Social Psychiatry* 4: 152-156, 1969.
13. FRANK J.: "The Dynamics of the Psychotherapeutic Relationship." *Psychiatry* 22: 17-34, 1959.
14. FRANK, J.: *Persuasion and Healing.* Baltimore: John Hopkins Press, 1961.
15. FREEMAN, H. AND SIMMONS, O.: *The Mental Patient Comes Home.* New York: Wiley, 1963.
16. GARFINKEL, H.: "Conditions of Successful Degradation Ceremonies." *American Journal of Sociology* 61: 420-424, 1956.
17. GARFINKEL, H.: "Some Conceptions of an Experiment with 'Trust' as a Condition of Stable Concerted Actions," in O. J. Harvey (ed.): *Motivation and Social Interaction.* New York: Ronald Press, 1963, Pp. 187-238.
18. GIBBS, J.: "Conceptions of Deviant Behavior: The Old and the New" *Pacific Sociological Review* 9: 9-14, 1966.
19. GOFFMAN, E.: *Asylums.* Garder City: Doubleday Anchor Books, 1961.
20. GOFFMAN, E.: *Stigma.* Englewood Cliffs: Prentice-Hall, 1963.
21. GOVE, W. R.: "Societal Reaction as an Explanation of Mental Illness." *American Sociological Review* 35: 873-883, 1970.
22. GUSFIELD, J. R.: "Moral Passage: The Symbolic Process in Public Designations of Deviance." *Social Problems* 15: 175-188, 1967.
23. HOLLINGSHEAD, A. B. AND REDLICH, F.: *Social Class and Mental Illness.* New York: Wiley, 1958.
24. HOROWITZ, I. L. AND LEIBOWITZ, M.: "Social Deviance and Political Marginality." *Social Problems* 15: 280-296, 1968.
25. LANGNER, T. S. AND MICHAEL, S. T.: *Life Stress and Mental Health: The Mid-Town Manhatten Study.* New York: Free Press, 1963.
26. LEMERT, E. M.: "Legal Commitment and Social Control." *Sociology and Social Research* 30: 370-378, 1946.
27. LEMERT, E. M.: *Human Deviance, Social Problems, and Social Control.* Englewood Cliffs: Prentice-Hall, 1967.
28. LEVINSON, D. J., AND GALLAGHER, E. B.: *Patienthood in the Mental Hospital.* Boston: Houghton Mifflin Company, 1964.
29. MESSINGER, S. L., SAMPSON, H., AND TOWNE, R. D.: "Life as Theater: Some Notes on the Dramaturgic Approach to Social Reality." *Sociometry* 25: 104, 1962.
30. MYERS, J. AND SCHAFFER, L.: "Social Stratification and Psychiatric Practice." *American Sociological Review* 19: 307-310, 1957.
31. PASAMANICK, B., et al.: *Schizophrenics in the Community.* New York: Appleton-Century-Crofts, 1967.
32. PERROW, C.: "Hospitals: Technology, Structure, and Goals," in James G. March (ed.): *Handbook of Organizations.* Chicago: Rand McNally and Company, Pp. 910-972.
33. QUINNEY, R. AND M. CLINARD. (eds.): *Criminal Behavior Systems.* New York: Holt, Rinehart, and Winston, 1967.
34. ROTH, J. A.: *Timetables.* Indianapolis: Bobbs-Merrill Company, 1963.
35. SAMPSON, H., MESSINGER, S. L., AND TOWNE, R. D.: "Family Processes and Becoming a Mental Patient." *American Journal of Sociology* 68: 88-96, 1962.
36. SAMPSON, H., MESSINGER, S. L., AND TOWNE, R. D.: *Schizophrenic Women: Studies in Marital Crises.* New York: Atherton, 1964.
37. SCHEFF, T. J.: *Being Mentally Ill: A Sociological Theory.* Chicago: Aldine Publishing Company, 1966.
38. SCHEFF, T. J. (ed.): *Mental Illness and Social Processes.* New York: Harper and Row, 1967.
39. SPIEGEL, J. P.: "The Social Roles of Doctor and Patient in Psychoanalysis and Psychotherapy." *Psychiatry* 17: 369-376, 1954.
40. SPITZER, S. AND DENZIN, N.: *The Mental Patient: Studies in Sociology of Deviance.* New York: McGraw-Hill, 1968.
41. STAR, S.: "The Public's Ideas about Mental Illness." Paper presented to National Association for Mental Health, Indianapolis, 1955.
42. STRAUSS, A., SCHATZMAN, L., EHRLICH, D., BUCHER, R., AND SABSHIN, M.: *Psychiatric Ideologies and Institutions.* New York: Free Press, 1964.

61

43. YARROW, M. R., SCHWARTZ, C. G., MURPHY, H. S., AND DEASY, L. C.: "The Psychological Meaning of Mental Illness in the Family." *Journal of Social Issues* 11: 12-24, 1955.
44. ZUBIN, J.: "Social Psychiatry and Psychopathology: A Layman's Comments on Contemporary Developments." Presented to the American Association for Psychopathology, New York, April, 1967.
45. GARFINKEL, H.: "Conditions of Successful Degradation Ceremonies." *American Journal of Sociology* 61: 420-424, 1956.
46. DENZIN, N. K.: "The Self-Fulfilling Prophecy and Patient-Therapist Interaction," in N. K. Denzin and S. Spitzer (eds.): *The Mental Patient: Studies in the Sociology of Deviance*. New York: McGraw Hill, 1968.

CHAPTER 4

The Search for Causes of Psychiatric Disorder*

LEE N. ROBINS

Our society increasingly recognizes a commitment to provide its citizens with environments which foster mental health and decrease risks of developing psychiatric disorder. Such a commitment demands increased knowledge of the specific social factors which contribute to psychiatric disorder as well as an understanding of their mechanisms of influence. At the present time, even if the finances and manpower to launch an ambitious program were available, we would be hard put to design a social environment that we could confidently expect to enhance the mental health of our society. Likewise, we would be hard put to decrease the rates of even a few of the psychiatric disorders that plague us.

Many sociological studies have sought to determine social causes of psychiatric disorder since Faris and Dunham first studied the relationship of demographic areas to psychiatric illness in 1939. Even though some correlations have been found to occur repeatedly, there have also been counter examples.[4] More importantly, there is good reason to question whether even the more regularly replicated results should be interpreted to mean that a certain social variable is the cause and the psychiatric disorder is the effect. Or is it at all clear, even if these correlations do imply cause, through what mechanisms social factors such as race, class, sex, and marital status affect rates of psychiatric disorder. Without knowing what the mechanisms are, policy decisions inevitably must be based more on hunches than on evidence about what changes are likely to be followed by a decrease in rates of disorder. For example, suppose that women do

*Supported by National Institute for Mental Health Research Scientist Award K5-MH-36-598, Research Grant MH-18864, and MH-13002. Revision of a paper presented to the Society for the Study of Social Problems, Washington, 1970.

experience a proportionately higher rate of psychiatric disorder than men, social programs designed to decrease these rates would have to be based on pure speculation about whether one or more of the many differences in sex roles in our society account for higher rates in women, or whether differential rates might result from suppositions concerned with lesser physical strength or biochemical makeup. Since there is no research evidence indicating *which* differences between men and women might be the culprits, one might equally well recommend that more women should hold jobs, take weight-lifting exercises, or try a dose of male hormones.

Our present lack of knowledge about the role of social factors involved in psychiatric disorders stems at least in part from methodological difficulties. In a previous paper,[16] I pointed to some of the difficulties inherent in demonstrating that a particular social correlate of a psychiatric disorder is more likely to be a cause of that disorder rather than its effect. A plea was made for 1) an accessibility to sample populations that were biased neither by socioeconomic status nor presence of psychiatric disorder, 2) demonstrating temporal priority by devoting attention to problems of dating the onset of disorder and events thought to have contributed to its appearance, 3) distinguishing symptoms from everyday problems in untreated samples, 4) working with objectively classified groups of affected persons, 5) recognition in sample design that familial correlates may reflect a common genetic predisposition rather than social effects, and 6) efforts to uncover the mechanisms through which a social correlate acts as a cause. Since the publication of that paper, we have continued to explore methods that would better achieve these goals. This chapter discusses some of the inadequacies present in the kinds of data we have been collecting. In addition, it will offer further innovative study designs which may provide greater confidence in our ability to identify social causes of psychiatric disorder and greater precision in describing their mechanisms of operation.

What most epidemiological studies of psychiatric disorder have attempted thus far, is to ascertain the frequency of psychiatric disorder in a population, divide that population along some social dimension, such as sex, age, or marital status, and then compare rates in one social category with those in another, such as males versus females, young versus old, or married versus unmarried.

Originally, such studies were done using hospitalized patients only. They compared proportions of women, Blacks, poor, and so forth among the hospitalized patients with proportions existing in the base population from which these patients were thought to come. Often the census was the source for such base rates. Critics pointed out a number of ways in which the results were biased. First, they were influenced by duration of hospitalization. This objection has been met by the use of incidence rates (first admission over a fixed interval) rather than prevalence rates (number of cases in treatment at a given time). This improvement does not, however, prevent bias created by the *duration of the disorder*. When services are differentially available by age group, geographic area, or social class, members of groups receiving less adequate services appear in a sample of first admissions only when their disorders are of long duration. If no facilities for adolescents are available, for instance, people with disorders during adolescence will appear in the sample only if that disorder persists into adulthood. Similarly, migrants to a city from areas with no treatment facilities who developed disorders prior to their migration will appear in a sample of first admissions only if the disorders persisted past the time of migration. If barriers to treatment are higher for one social class than another, transient disorders will appear in a sample of first admissions only for those who have easier access to treatment. The *duration of the disorder* can thus bias its appearance in a treated sample even when the use of incidence rates, rather than prevalence rates, prevents the *duration of treatment* variable from affecting rates.

Additionally the results were biased by social status differences in seeking and being accepted for professional care, by more adequate reporting of public than of private facilities, by social bias in the assignment of diagnostic labels, and by differences in residential mobility in the geographic area from which patients came which made the census estimates of the base population inappropriate, because some areas had relatively enormous turnovers of population and changes in the character of the population over the time of the study.

To meet these criticisms, studies were moved into the residential community, where they attempted to locate all cases of psychiatric disturbance in a given area over a brief period of time. The change from hospital to community studies corrected the bias engendered by differences in the likelihood of the patient coming for treatment and in the completeness with which various types of treatment facilities were covered, in length of hospital stay, and in residential area turnover. The application of uniform criteria for psychiatric disturbance, regardless of social background, avoided class-biased diagnosis. Thus, the chief criticisms leveled against hospital studies were met. Two important new problems were added—that of establishing criteria for what constituted a psychiatric case and of deciding to which category of psychiatric disorder it belonged. These difficulties have seriously compromised the advantages of the area survey. Even more importantly, the area survey continued to suffer from other problems which had existed in hospital studies, but had been less widely acknowledged.

Both hospital and area surveys have gathered data concerning *current* rates of psychiatric disorder within *current* social categories. But identifying probable social causes requires more than establishing degrees of correlations between psychiatric disorders and social factors. First, it requires establishing temporal priority of the presumed cause over the presumed outcome; in other words, what we need to know before considering a social variable a probable cause of psychiatric disorder is that membership in one social category is more likely to be *followed* by the onset of psychiatric disorder than is membership in another. Since social factors such as occupational and marital status, and geographic location may be influenced by the psychiatric disorder, we cannot assume that current social category memberships predated the disorder or were independent of it. We must then identify the social category memberships *prior* to the onset of psychiatric disorder.

Second, we must learn whether psychiatric disorder followed membership in a social category at *any* later date, not whether it was present at a particular moment. Psychiatric disorders have onsets at widely varying ages (from under two years of age for infantile autism to over seventy for senility) and they differ greatly in their likelihood of remission (from chronic brain syndromes which virtually never remit, through depressions and manias which usually last only a few months, to acute toxic psychoses which may last only a few hours). Rarely have studies of treated population samples or area surveys provided estimates of risks of disorder over the entire life-span following membership in a social category. Some of the Scandinavian and German studies[7, 9, 20] have recognized the need for estimating the risks over a lifetime for general populations and have developed methods of calculating such risks, but they have not been able to cope with the problem of ascertaining whether membership in a social category preceded the onset of psychiatric disorder. Helgason[8] brilliantly discusses the need for such methods. American studies, however, have show little awareness of the necessity for estimates of risk over a lifetime. Most of our studies of psychiatric disorder in a general population sample have asked questions like "Are you the worrying type?" or "Are you often troubled by shortness of breath?" The answers to such questions give estimates only of the prevalence of any given disorder at the moment of interview or within some brief time span selected by the respondent as defining "the present." Studies of prevalence in area surveys, such as hospitals, may tend to primarily identify those disorders which are characterized by early onset and chronicity, because these disorders have appeared before and persisted until the time of interview. On the other hand, those psychiatric disorders which are characterized by remission or late onset are likely to be missed.

The study of social causes of psychiatric disorder requires not only showing that the social factor occurred first and was at some time followed by psychiatric disorder, but also that "other things were equal" between the two groups. One of the important ways in which "other things" may *not* be equal is in the number of years during which persons with and without the social variable are at risk. The third requirement for identifying a social cause is that it is followed by disorder more frequently than expected, given an equal exposure to risk. The exposure to risk must be equal not only in *length* of time but also in age span, since various psychiatric disorders are characterized by distinctive periods of onset. Amark,[1] for instance, has shown that in a Scandinavian population virtually no one experiences alcohol problems for the first time after age 50. Therefore, we would almost certainly find a low incidence of alcoholism among the widowed, but we should *not* conclude that widowhood protects against alcoholism. We must either compare groups exposed at the same ages or statistically compensate for differences.

66

Other important ways in which social groups may differ are in their rates of physical illness or in the degree of genetic predisposition to psychiatric disorder. Physical illness is more common among the aged, for example, and can lead both to conditions of social isolation and to changes in the brain which are reflected in the confusion and memory loss typical of chronic brain syndrome. Conditions of social isolation may appear earlier than the symptoms of confusion, and so predate the psychiatric problems, but the psychiatric problems would have been as likely to occur even in the absence of social isolation. Similarly, ethnic groups and geographic enclaves tend to be endogamous and thus to share genetic pools. The problem of differentiating genetic from social factors is particularly difficult in studying the "under the roof" culture of the family as the social variable of interest. The mode of transmission of the disorder from the parent to child might be entirely genetic; yet the symptoms of the parent's disorder will play a role in determining the kind of social environment in which the child is reared. If the parent is paranoid, for example, his suspiciousness and hostility are likely to alienate relatives and neighbors, resulting in an absence of ordinary opportunities for his child to learn normal patterns of social interaction. If the child himself then grows up exhibiting suspicious and hostile patterns of behavior, we need to find out whether this is fully explained by the genetic contribution of the paranoid parent, or whether his abnormal rearing has played a part. To determine whether a social hypothesis is more plausible than a physical illness or genetic hypothesis, medical and family histories of psychiatric disorder must be obtained. If we suspect that a particular social factor may be associated with increased rates of psychiatric disorder for people *without* a history of preexisting physical illness and *without* parents who exhibit symptoms of the same disorder, we are increasingly convinced that it has indeed played a role in the onset of disorder.

If we are to determine the social causes of psychiatric disorder and their mechanisms of action, we need then to work on these methodological problems:

1) Obtaining unbiased samples of persons with known social factors prior to the onset of disorder
2) Obtaining life-span estimates for the development of psychiatric disorders subsequent to their social category membership
3) Equalizing the age-span during which those with and without the social factor are at risk
4) Ruling out competing causal hypotheses, such as physical disease or genetic predisposition
5) Investigating what the mechanisms of operation may be for those social factors that survive these requirements as plausibly causal.

The remainder of the chapter will discuss some methods that hopefully will improve our abilities to tackle these five goals.

CHOOSING POPULATION SAMPLES ON THE BASIS
OF SOCIAL VARIABLES PREDATING THE ONSET
OF PSYCHIATRIC DISORDER

A universally recognized criterion for a plausible cause is that an event has occurred before its presumed effect. Equally important, but less commonly stated, is the requirement that determining the presence or absence of that hypothetical cause must not be biased by the occurrence of the later event that we would like to show as the effect. There is no danger of such bias if, in seeking social causes of psychiatric disorder, we choose a sample of persons both with and without a social characteristic *before* any of them have any psychiatric disorder, patiently follow them through the period of risk, and then examine them to see whether they have developed a psychiatric disorder. We may then legitimately compare rates of disorder between persons who originally did and did not have the social variable. In practice, however, studies are often done in reverse order, choosing samples in which some persons already have a psychiatric disorder and inquiring retrospectively about their social characteristics prior to the onset of disorder. A significantly higher rate of an early occurring social characteristic in the ill than in the well is then interpreted to mean that the social characteristic may be a cause, since it is both correlated with the disorder and occurred prior to it. Such an inference may not be justified.

Consider that a study, which attempts to discover the degree of correlation between the size of an individual's hometown and incidence of psychiatric disorder, is carried out in a sleepy backwater town undergoing rapid transition to a city as a result of new industry. Suppose that when a random sample is queried regarding psychiatric disorder and place of upbringing, we find that those brought up in small towns have the highest rate of psychiatric disorder. There is a very plausible alternative to the hypothesis that small towns are detrimental to mental health. Many individuals in our small-town-reared sample will have been born in the very town in which they now live as adults, and will have remained here throughout the period when there was little economic opportunity. Stability of residence when local opportunity is poor may often be a consequence of psychiatric disorder. The sample population reared on farms and in cities, on the other hand, are by definition all in-migrants to the town, who may well be a healthier-than-average group attracted there by the new industry. We therefore have a small town sample possibly biased in the direction of psychiatric disorder and city and farm samples biased in the direction of psychiatric health. Similar possibilities of bias apply to all studies of adults in restricted geographic areas. In a highly mobile society such as ours, place of residence is a function of capability and health. The old resident in a declining neighborhood may remain there because he is psychiatrically, intellectually, or physically disabled; the new resident may come because he is a healthier-than-average upwardly mobile person from the slum or ghetto. In surveys of restricted geographic areas, inferences about the psychiatric effects of race or social status of the childhood home are thus confounded by the differing meaning of residence in such an area to persons of divergent backgrounds.

The bias that place of residence introduces into the probability of finding psychiatric disorder in one social group as compared with another can be avoided by utilizing studies that evaluate prior social variables retrospectively by studying either a total society or a geographically isolated community, since in both cases in and out migration is trivial. It can also be avoided by choosing a sample population young enough so that the place of residence is not determined by the subject himself, and thus cannot be influenced by his psychiatric disorder. Following a sample of children thus selected until they have passed the risk period for psychiatric disorder, however, necessitates a long delay in completing the study. Alternatively, we can select our follow-up sample from old records such as birth or school records, which were made before any psychiatric disability occurred and made long enough ago so that the sample population has already had time to develop psychiatric disorder. Then we can complete the follow-up immediately, locating members of the sample population wherever they live as adults and learning from interview or early records their place of upbringing, race, or childhood social class, or whatever other social variables that existed prior to the onset of psychiatric disorder in which we are interested in. We can then be sure that our samples of people with and without this social characteristic have not been biased by their later geographic location and thus by the psychiatric disorder which is our dependent variable.

If a follow-up study seems too difficult, even when no waiting period is involved, and if a study of a total society is unwieldy or an isolated area inappropriate to the question raised, the best compromise seems to be to select residential areas in which mobility is minimal and then to *discard* the few mobile cases so that the sample is uniform with respect both to place of birth and current residence. To study the influence of a factor such as place of rearing, one would then have to use multiple sampling areas. The drawback in studying only immobile samples is that the effect of a variable such as class or race can then be generalized only to immobile populations.

Before accepting such a compromise, it is well to consider the many advantages the follow-up study offers in addition to providing population samples unbiased by later psychiatric disorder. One such advantage is the ability to develop a system of stratification on the social variable to be investigated. Because early records, from which the follow-up sample is selected, often provide information about sex, race, address, and parents' names, we may be able to use these as indicators of the social variable in which we are interested and thus choose approximately equal groups both with and without the social characteristic. For a fixed sample size, having equal-sized subgroups maximizes our ability to detect the effect of the subgroup characteristic on psychiatric status. Thus follow-up studies provide efficient as well as unbiased samples. The sample can be made still more efficient by using as control variables indicators in the early records of other social factors that might contaminate our findings (ensuring, for instance, that we have equal numbers of males and females within each social class stratum). Sampling from early records also permits choosing samples in which all persons involved are approximately the same age so that they all will have the same number of years at risk of experiencing psychiatric disorder.

In addition, and perhaps most important, a follow-up study provides a more accurate count of the affected persons and more accurate comparisons of the effects of the social variable than does a cross-sectional study. Since the follow-up study provides us with a list of people to be accounted for, we must attempt to trace even those persons who are hard to find at home, transient, imprisoned, or dead; all groups which are likely to contain more than the usual share of psychiatric disorder. Cross-sectional studies, with no master list even of persons alive at a given point in time, are particularly likely to miss (1) persons with antisocial personality, alcoholism, and drug addiction problems because of the association of these disorders with transiency, imprisonment, hospitalization, and early death; (2) persons with a history of severe depression, because this disorder has a high suicide risk; and (3) cases of chronic brain syndrome because again there is both a high death rate and a high rate of long-term hospitalization. Missed cases in cross-sectional studies cause not only underestimates of rates of those disorders associated with inaccessibility and early death, but also an *exaggeration* of the differences in the rates of these disorders between social groups. As the loss of cases decreases the percentage of cases discovered, it increases the ratio between these percentages. For example, suppose 40 per cent of Group A and 20 per cent of Group B actually develop a particular set of psychiatric disorders, a ratio of 2.0:1. Next suppose that a cross-sectional study is biased only by the loss of half of the people with these disorders. The loss reduces the rate of disorder in Group A to 25 per cent $[40 - 1/2 (40)$ divided by $100 - 1/2 (40)]$ and in Group B to 11 per cent $[20 - 1/2 (20)$ divided by $100 - 1/2 (20)]$. The ratio between the percentages with disorder in the two groups *increases* to 2.3:1.

Whether one chooses follow-up techniques or cross-sectional samples of stable populations or total societies, the yield of individuals with a given psychiatric disorder will be a small proportion of the total sample. When one wants to study social factors contributing to a specific disorder, this small yield makes both longitudinal and cross-sectional studies of general populations unsatisfactory. Instead, we need methods for identifying high-risk populations, in order to get enough affected cases. To define a high-risk population requires knowing something about how the disorder is distributed in the population, even if one does not know whether its correlates are in any sense causes of the disorder. If one knows the sex and age distribution of the disorder or that it tends to run in families, one can sample from populations in which it occurs frequently.

While providing adequate numbers of cases, sampling from high-risk populations has two drawbacks. First, the variable (age, sex, or family history) used to locate the high-risk population is lost as a possible cause, because it will have occurred in every case, in both those with and those without the disorder. Second, what we find about social variables correlated with and preceding the disorder applies only to this subsample of the total population. In studying social factors in alcoholism, for example, if we sample only men because their alcoholism rate is 3 to 5 times higher than women's, and if we then find that broken homes predict alcoholism, we still will not know whether broken homes predict *female* alcoholism nor *why* men are more prone to alcoholism than women. What we would like is a way of identifying a high-risk population which provides a sample representative of the total population with that disorder. We would then be free to study any social variable as a potential cause and could generalize our findings to the whole population of affected persons.

We are currently exploring a method that we hope will accomplish this, at least for certain disorders. We noted in the course of a follow-up study in which I obtained both interview and record information, that men identified by interview as alcoholics could be so identified in records alone in only 25 per cent of the cases,[15] but that they did have patterns of record appearance that were somewhat distinctive. Alcoholics had more arrests late in life (whether or not associated with drinking problems), more arrests for a property offense, more hospitalizations for a variety of reasons, more treatment for injury, more reports as absence without leave while in the service, more failure to finish high school, and more poor credit ratings. We have been exploring ways of choosing patterns of record appearance that yield a sample of alcoholics unbiased with respect to social status and other social variables and which select as few nonalcoholics as possible. We will then test the pattern of records found most efficient in selecting a representative sample of subjects identified as alcoholic during an interview in additional samples of Whites and Blacks, men and women, from St. Louis and San Francisco to learn whether it continues to be efficient and unbiased for various kinds of populations.

If a representative high-risk sample can be chosen from records, one would then have to locate members of the sample population and establish through interview which members are alcoholic and their social history prior to becoming so. A control group of nonalcoholics for comparison with the alcoholics thus identified could be selected from persons residing in the areas the alcoholics had lived in before their drinking problems began. The "negatives" in the high-risk population are *not* an appropriate control group because we have no reason to believe that a sample of persons with records similar to alcoholics who are not alcoholics represent any kind of normal sample. Indeed, we suspect they may be pre-alcoholics. Similar methods, using different record criteria, probably can be developed for selecting samples with high risk of some other psychiatric syndromes as well.

Obtaining Estimates for the Development of Psychiatric Disorder

When researchers moved from treated samples to the field, they had to face the problem of who should be counted as having a psychiatric disorder and what disorder he should be counted as having. Actually, the problem had existed in treated samples as well. While the official diagnosis was usually accepted, the official assignment to one diagnostic category rather than another was likely to be erratic in the present state of American psychiatry. Even in countries where there is more agreement about nomenclature or in American hospitals where there is a common interest in diagnosis and a common training in definitions, the official diagnosis seldom meets research criteria for uniform data collection and decision rules. Even the assumption that everyone who is being treated has *some* disorder can be challenged in those communities where psychiatrists are perceived as the professionals of choice to consult about marital difficulties or as educators in self-acceptance.

Baffled by the lack of unanimity among American psychiatrists about the meaning of diagnostic terms and by their lack of interest in categorizing patients, field researchers have used degree of severity, "caseness," and impairment as their criteria rather than a diagnostic nomenclature. Despite the obvious problems with current diagnostic schemes, some attention to diagnostic categories seems necessary. Every study using diagnostic categories, no matter how crude, has found marked differences in their social correlates. Childhood behavior disorders, alcoholism, drug addiction, mental defect, and antisocial personality are found predominantly among poor men; some neuroses and depression predominate among women and are either uncorrelated with social class or more common in the middle class; schizophrenia is found equally among the two sexes but predominates among the lower class and the young. These correlates have been found in studies conducted with many kinds of samples and in various countries.*

Such substantial correlations strongly suggest that if social variables are causal, they must be specific to particular disorders. We suspect that social correlates have been found in field studies which lumped all psychiatric disorder together only because the instruments used were sensitive only to certain kinds of disorder. It seems probable, for instance, that the repeated findings in area surveys of an association of a particular psychiatric disorder with women and increasing age can be attributed to the fact that the interviews have emphasized symptoms of depression and hysteria and the subjective experience of poor physical health. Depression and hysteria are predominant in women; poor physical health in the elderly. These interview schedules almost totally omitted questions about behavior disorders, alcoholism, and drug addiction, which are disorders with early onsets, amelioration after middle age, and have a predominance in men.

---

*An exhaustive bibliography of the social correlates of psychiatric disorder is beyond the scope of this chapter. Some particularly useful sources are, for all disorders: Rosen and associates;[18] Malzberg;[12] Helgason;[8] for drug addiction: Larimore and Brill;[11] O'Donnell;[13] for alcoholism: Cahalan;[3] Knupfer;[10] for childhood disorders: Rutler;[19] for mental defect: Douglas;[5] for antisocial personality: Robins.[14]

If we are to be able to ascertain rates of particular disorders, we must ask sufficient questions about each symptom of the disorders in which we are interested to detect or rule out its presence. Since we are interested in a lifetime history of disorder, we must know whether at any previous period in time the subject would have qualified as having the disorder. This means that symptom questions must be phrased as "have you ever—," not "do you—." Positive answers must be followed by questions about when the event occurred, for how long, and how severe it was. The reason for these requirements is that a psychiatric syndrome is ordinarily defined by a set of sensations and/or behaviors occurring *together* which are more frequent, more persistent, and more severe, but not necessarily qualitatively different, than the experience of people without the syndrome. The questions usually asked in previous studies have only established the presence or absence of a symptom without sufficient information to classify it as being different from ordinary experiences of life stress nor as concurrent with other symptoms in a syndrome rather than isolated.

The development of comprehensive psychiatric registers[2] promises to be of great assistance in developing lifetime histories of disorder. Supplementing interviews with register data should help compensate for the fact that the recent and more severe disorders are more likely to be recalled in interview[14] than are more earlier and milder disorders.

We suggested above that past efforts at discovering psychiatric disorder have concentrated particularly on the neuroses and on depression. These are disorders which are not only easy to inquire about without embarrassing the subject or the interviewer, but are also disorders that can be established exclusively by personal interview, since the primary symptoms are internal distress. This is not true of all psychiatric disorders. For some, an interview with the subject is less useful— young children, stuporous psychotic patients, and paranoid patients whose coherent and plausible story of persecution defies skepticism are examples. One needs outside information from relatives or hospital records in such cases. In other syndromes, such as those involving the drug addict or alcoholic, the interview is essential, but because of the danger of dissembling and poor memory for chronological detail, outside verification as well is advisable.

Disorders also differ in the ideal age at which to obtain information. Because we would like a lifetime history, one might think the ideal subject is very old, since he will have passed through the age of risk of all disorders. The danger is that by the time his whereabouts had been located he may have died, and those disorders that require personal interviews would be missed. In addition, many disorders ameliorate or totally disappear with time. An elderly person may well have forgotten his childhood behavior disorder, and no parent would have survived to serve as an outside informant. Ideally, each disorder should be studied in persons who have recently passed through the age of risk for onset of that disorder. Thus, all cases that will ever occur will have occurred, and the disorder will either still be present or easily remembered because it is recent. In practice, one can only approximately fulfill such a goal. Yet some restriction in the age range and adjustment by weighting for persons not yet through the period of risk would be an improvement over current practices of interviewing people of widely varying ages, such as 20 to 59.

Since various disorders require different sources of information and different ages at investigation, it is probably a mistake to try to cover the total spectrum of psychiatric disorder in a single study. One would do better to group together those disorders which have common ages of onset and which need the same kind of evidence. For disorders such as depression, with onsets over a wide age-range and with such brief episodes that the chance of being forgotten is great, one would need individuals of different ages. After asking such a sample population about episodes of depression in the last 10 years prior to interview, an estimate for lifetime risk can be calculated by drawing a composite portrait of the risk of depression in each age period.

Equalizing Time Spans for Psychiatric Disorder

Many of the variables in which we have been interested as possible social causes are determined at birth: sex, race, and place of birth. Present from birth, they are inevitably also present when the subject enters the period of risk for developing any particular psychiatric disorder. Other social variables, however, first occur after some of the period of risk has already passed. Marriage is an example of such a variable. How then are we to interpret the fact that those suffering from schizophrenic disorder are infrequently married? One possibility is that having a serious psychiatric disorder makes it unlikely that a person will marry, both because he is unattractive to others and because he has little interest in finding a spouse. Conversely, it is also possible in theory that marriage somehow protects individuals against schizophrenia. Exploring this hypothesis, we note that by the time most people marry, they have already passed through about half the age of risk for ever developing schizophrenia (assuming the risk period is approximately between the ages of 16 and 35). If we were to choose a sample of children and follow them past the age of risk for schizophrenia, counting as cases in which being single may contribute to schizophrenia and those cases in which marriage may contribute to schizophrenia, we would find a higher rate of schizophrenia among singles than among married people even if marriage did *not* protect against schizophrenia, because the state of being single begins at birth and the state of being married only about age 20. To argue that marriage protects one from schizophrenia, we need to compare married and unmarried persons at risk for the same length of time and during the identical age-span. That is, we cannot compensate for the later exposure to risk of the married by following them an additional 20 years, because the they would be studied at ages with a different vulnerability to schizophrenia than would the singles. The solution to this problem seems to be a statistical one. We need to apply to our data the kinds of actuarial methods of analysis that are used in the "combined-risk life table" that insurance companies use to decide whether and at what ages bachelors have a greater risk of death than married men. We can substitute our measures of psychiatric disorder for the death variable and the onset of any social variable not present at birth in place of the marriage variable. We have tried such a technique in investigating predictors of drug use.[17] We developed a computer program that counts each person as being without the social variable (that is, single) up to the age at which he marries or develops the disorder, transfers him to the group with the social variable (that is, those who are married), when that variable occurs if he is still free of disorder at that time, and then age-adjusts the group without the social variable still at risk of disorder (the healthy single individuals) to the ages of persons with the predictor variable still at risk of disorder (the healthy married individuals) before computing rates of disorder for the two groups.

This method can be applied only when the age of first entering risk (for example, age at marriage) and the age of onset of disorder are both known. To equalize time spans at risk, we must, therefore, collect data not only concerning which social variables preceded disorders but also at what age the social variable was first experienced and at what age the first symptoms of disorder appeared. It is immediately apparent that such dating is not possible for disorders with insidious onset. For such disorders, only social variables present at birth can unequivocally be shown to predate them. While social variables that occurred later may also be causal, there will always be some doubt about whether such a variable is more probably a cause or more probably an effect of the disorder.

Ruling Out Physical and Genetic Explanations in Psychiatric Disorder

When a subject has a physical illness, it is difficult to assess whether the illness explains all his symptoms or whether he may not simultaneously have a psychiatric disorder. In young people, serious illness is sufficiently rare so that the only necessary precaution is to ask for a medical history and discard those cases in which the picture is confused by illness. Similar practice in studies of the elderly involves much greater sample losses, but we have not yet found a way to separate physical from social causes of disorder other than by excluding those claiming physical illness. This is clearly an unsatisfactory situation, since a delusion of illness can be a symptom of psychiatric disorder and since medical and psychiatric disorders can exist simultaneously. One can perhaps find solace in realizing that this same perplexity faces the psychiatrist trying to make a diagnosis in a patient for whom he has abundant laboratory data. Even normal laboratory tests do not rule out the possibility of undetected physical disease nor does a positive physical finding rule out simultaneous and independent psychiatric disorder.

To distinguish social from genetic explanations, one must inquire about the family history of psychiatric disorder. Those cases whose parents had the disorder in which we are interested are then treated as a separate group in further analysis. One would not want to discard cases with a possible genetic component, as we suggested doing for physical disorders, because we would then miss the opportunity to identify the social factors which may trigger the disorders in persons with a genetic predisposition.

The segregation of those with and without a suspected genetic component serves nicely to decide whether factors such as social class, family size, and broken homes (which may themselves be determined by the parental disorders) are more likely mere correlates of the parent's disorder or contribute directly to the risk of disorder in the child. But when the social variable to be investigated is the parental disorder itself, obviously no segregation by a suspected genetic variable is possible. One would have to compare rates in a sample whose parents have the disorder with rates in a sample whose parents do not have the disorder yet have the same genetic background—a clearly impossible task. Still the parental disorder might be a social variable, influencing the child by parental example or by creating a family environment which in turn fosters the same disorder. On the other hand, the parental disorder might equally well reflect a genetic variable at work or account for an abnormal prenatal physical environment, if for example a depressed mother failed to eat adequately during her pregnancy. To find out whether the parental disorder operates as a social variable, rather than genetically or by changing the intrauterine environment, one must employ one of two natural experiments: adoption, where the social parents are not the biological ones, or twinning, where monozygotic and dizygotic twins differ in the proportion of shared genes but minimally in intrauterine and later environments. Monozygotic twins, in fact, have more different intrauterine environments than do dizygotic twins. Therefore, a greater concordance in disorders between monozygotic twins is an especially strong argument for a genetic factor. If this approach is not taken one must expand the family history questions during interviews to obtain complete pedigrees of disorder with ages of both affected and unaffected family members to provide the data necessary to test whether familial rates of disorder are consistent with genetic formulae. In sum, ordinary surveys will not tell us whether psychiatric disorder in the parents is a *social* determinant of the same disorder in their offspring.

Investigating Mechanisms for Operation of Social Variables

Once we have identified a social factor that predates a specific psychiatric disorder, that remains correlated with it when age at risk is taken into account, and that cannot be explained away as a result of physical illness or as a consequence of the same disorder in the parent or as the correlate of some other social factor, we have met all the tests for its plausibility as a cause of the disorder. Yet until we know through what mechanisms it operates, we will not be able to plan any action that can be expected to reduce the rate of disorder. The search for mechanisms is important not only because of its practical applications, but is also essential if we are to develop further a theoretical understanding of how society shapes human behavior and human psychological experience.

A mechanism through which a social variable contributes to psychiatric disorder is correlated with both the social variable and the disorder and occurs prior to the onset of the disorder. When the mechanism is absent, the level of correlation between the social factor and the social disorder is reduced. As an example of a possible mechanism, consider the hypothesis that the low rate of alcoholism among Italians is explained by their custom of introducing children to drinking as part of family mealtime ritual. This custom is thought to divest drinking of the secular, euphoric connotations that it has for the Irish male. Given that being Italian protects one against alcoholism and being Irish predisposes one to alcoholism, we must design our research to help us decide whether the meaning Italians attribute to drinking through the socialization of children to drinking is a more probable mechanism than a number of others one might suggest, such as differences in the choice of beverages (wine *versus* whisky), the frequency of drinking on an empty stomach, or the customary amount drunk per hour in a drinking session, to name only a few. We fail to produce evidence for one mechanism in preference to another so long as we continue merely to catalog differences between Italian and Irish cultures both with respect to drinking behavior and in other ways. Instead, we must compare the customs and values of alcoholics and nonalcoholics *within* the Irish community and *within* the Italian community. If we find that nonalcoholic Irishmen were much more often introduced to whisky at family meals than at the tavern, while for alcoholic Irishmen it was the reverse, we substantiate the hypothesis that the Italian way of educating their children to drink may be the mechanism. On the other hand, if alcoholic and nonalcoholic Irishmen both began drinking in the tavern, but the nonalcoholics hated the taste of whisky and so drank beer or wine, we would favor the choice-of-beverage hypothesis.

To learn the mechanisms through which a social variable operates, interviews should include not only the questions about demographic data ordinarily used to establish social group membership, but also questions allowing a test of all the major hypotheses that would explain *why* one social group differs from another in rates of disorder. We would then be prepared to discard as possible mechanisms those variables which did not distinguish alcoholics from nonalcoholics *within* an ethnic group, and to suggest as worthy of experimentation policies which might engender those behaviors, tastes, and attitudes which are associated with low rates of disorder within susceptible groups.

If the mechanism of action of a social variable like ethnicity turns out to be biochemical (as the effect of whisky compared to the effect of wine would be) rather than a more psychological mechanism (such as attitudes toward alcohol or drunkenness), we should not feel that our work is any less sociological. Certainly dietary choices are as much socially determined as is the manner of socializing children to drinking. Nor is the design of a useful social policy more difficult if the mechanism *is* biochemical. Given our current high development of advertising skills, changing drinkers' preferences for a beverage, and thus their exposure to a biochemical agent, should be at least as feasible as persuading Bible Belt parents to serve wine with meals.

CONCLUSIONS

Social policy likely to reduce rates of new cases of psychiatric disorder must be based on a knowledge of the social causes of psychiatric disorder and the mechanisms through which these social factors operate. This chapter suggests some innovations which might improve our certainty (1) that the hypothetical social cause preceded the disorder, (2) that the samples of persons with and without the social variable are not biased with respect to later disorder, (3) that persons with and without the hypothetical social cause had the same age-spans at the risk of disorder, (4) that we have accurately determined the presence and kind of psychiatric disorder over the whole period at risk, (5) that the correlation between the presumed social cause and the psychiatric disorder was not the spurious effect of physical illness or genetic predisposition, and (6) that we learn the nature of the mechanisms through which the social determinant appears to act.

To accomplish these goals a number of innovations have been suggested in samples to be used, questionnaire design, use of records and outside informants, and statistical analysis. These suggestions stem from a conviction that we have gone as far as we can with static demographic descriptions of the distribution of undifferentiated psychiatric disorder as the source of hypotheses about the social causes of psychiatric disorder. Probably many of the hypotheses we have thus derived are correct. To find out *which* ones are, we need studies based on unbiased samples, studies carefully designed to show relationships among specified social variables, their mechanisms of action, and carefully delineated psychiatric disorders, holding constant competing variables. The samples and methods should be chosen for their appropriateness to the particular disorder to be investigated and to the specific hypothesis about its causes to be tested, because we cannot fruitfully investigate all disorders and all causes simultaneously.

When we base policy suggestions on demonstrations that our hypothetical causal variables preceded specific psychiatric disorders in unbiased samples, despite corrections for genetic and physical factors and years at risk, and when we can show the intervening variables between these social variables and disorder, our suggestions for social policy aimed at decreasing rates of those particular psychiatric disorders will be as enlightened as nonexperimental studies can make them. Enactment of the policies we suggest in limited areas can then provide the crucial experiment to test the correctness of our causal hypotheses by comparing rates of new disorder within the experimental area with rates in matched areas where the policy has not been enacted.

REFERENCES

1. AMARK, C.: "A Study of Alcoholism." *Acta Psychiatrica et Neurologicia Scandanavia,* Suppl. 70, 1951.
2. BAHN, A. K.: "A New Psychiatric Epidemiology." *Israel Annals of Psychiatry* 2:11-18, 1964.
3. CAHALAN, D.: *Problem Drinking.* San Francisco: Jossey-Bass, 1970.
4. DOHRENWEND, B. P., AND DOHRENWEND, B. S.: *Social Status and Psychological Disorder.* Chapter 2. New York: Wiley-Interscience, 1969.
5. DOUGLAS, J. W. B.: *The Home and School.* London: MacGibbon & Kee, 1964.
6. FARIS, R. E. L., AND DUNHAM, H. W.: *Mental Disorders in Urban Areas.* Chicago: University of Chicago Press, 1939.
7. FREMMING, K. H.: "The Expectation of Mental Infirmity in a Sample of Danish Population." Occasional Papers on Eugenics No. 7. Eugenics Society and Cassell & Co., Ltd., 1951.
8. HELGASON, T.: *Epidemiology of Mental Disorders in Iceland.* Copenhagen: Munksgaard, 1964.
9. KLEMPERER, J.: "Zur Belastungsstatistik der Durchschnittsbevölkerung." *Z. ges Neurolog. Psychiatrica* 146:277-316, 1933.
10. KNUPFER, G.: "The Epidemiology of Problem Drinking." *American Journal of Public Health* 57:973-986, 1967.
11. LARIMORE, G. W., AND BRILL, H.: "Epidemiologic Factors in Drug Addiction in England and the United States." *Public Health Reports* 77:555-560, 1962.
12. MALZBERG, B.: *The Mental Health of the Negro.* Albany, New York: Research Foundation for Mental Hygiene, Inc., 1963.
13. O'DONNELL, J. A.: "Social Factors and Follow-up Studies in Opioid Addiction." in the *The Addictive States.* Baltimore: Williams and Wilkins, 1968, pp. 333-346, 1968.
14. ROBINS, L. N.: *Deviant Children Grown Up.* Baltimore: Williams & Wilkins, 1966.
15. ROBINS, L. N., MURPHY, G. E., AND BRECKENRIDGE, M. B.: "Drinking behaviour of young urban Negro men." *Quarterly Journal of Studies on Alcohol* 29:657-684, 1968.
16. ROBINS, L. N.: "Social Correlates of Psychiatric Disorders: Can We Tell Causes from Consequences?" *Journal of Health and Social Behaviour* 10:95-104, 1969.
17. ROBINS, L. N., AND TAIBELSON, M.: "An Actuarial Method for Assessing the Direction of Influence Between Datable Life Events." *Sociological Methods and Research* 1:243-270, 1971.
18. ROSEN, B. M., BAHN, A. K., AND KRAMER, M.: "Demographic and diagnostic characteristics of Psychiatric Clinics Outpatients in the U.S.A." *American Journal of Orthopsychiatry* 34:455-468, 1964.
19. RUTLER, M. L.: "Psycho-social Disorders in Childhood and Their Outcome in Adult Life." *Journal of the Royal College of Physicians* (London) 4:211-218, 1970.
20. STRONIGREN, T.: "Beitrage zur Psychiatrischen Erblehre." *Acta Psychiatrica Scandanavia* Suppl. 19, 1938.

CHAPTER 5

Problems of Cross-Cultural Research in Psychiatric Sociology*

CONSTANTINA SAFILIOS-ROTHSCHILD
AND MICHAEL MOORE

The methodological problems involved in cross-cultural research in psychiatric sociology fall into two categories: those common to all cross-cultural sociological research regardless of the subject, and those due to the present state of sociology in any country. In other words, while some methodological problems arise only when cross-cultural investigations are undertaken, others exist simply because the state of the scientific inquiry in a particular field is not satisfactory in any country. Whenever serious measurement problems and shortcomings exist in a field, even in the countries in which this field is most developed, cross-cultural research simply multiplies and exaggerates the existing problems.

In this chapter we first examine some general methodological problems involved in all cross-cultural research and then turn to problems more specifically relevant to research in psychiatric sociology.

GENERAL METHODOLOGICAL PROBLEMS†

Availability of Research Staff

The degree of comparability of research data gathered cross-culturally depends to a considerable extent not only upon the degree of comparability of the

*Sincere thanks are due to Drs. E. D. Wittkower, R. Prince, and F. Engelsmann of the Section of Transcultural Psychiatric Studies at McGill University for their comments and suggestions to an earlier draft of this chapter.

†Some of the material for the section on "General Methodological Proglems" has been taken from the authors' joint working paper on "Methodological Issues in Cross-Cultural Research," written for the Cross-National Family Studies Project supported by a subcontract PH-43-68-972 with Case Western Reserve University.

81

research techniques used and the questions asked but also upon the degree of similarity in the training and abilities of interviewers and other field research assistants. The latter factor, however, has not up to now received the degree of attention that it merits. Researchers tend to use any type of interviewer and field assistant that is available in each social and cultural setting. Sometimes, however, amateurs such as social workers, school teachers, and college students have been used with considerable success, although this practice is strongly opposed by some investigators.[59] In most developing countries, interviewing and other field work is usually underpaid and sporadic work because of the scarcity of research projects. Since there are not many or in some cases any sociology or psychology graduate students who would be doing this kind of work as part of their professional training and experience, there is usually no regular, well-trained, and experienced pool of interviewers and field workers available. As a result each investigator must locate potential staff, train them, and motivate them to stay on. Because of the very marginal status of such work in most developing countries, those who undertake it are either between jobs or have already stable and regular job employment, facts which lessen their commitment to their field work. Due to the low degree of work commitment that places this type of work last in the hierarchy of their preoccupations, one usually has to train four or five times as many people as he needs in order to have the necessary staff.[68] Some investigators have found that the investigator-interviewer relationship was satisfactory and enduring only when it was based on personal "sympathy" and loyalty,[68] close personal contact providing supervision as well as moral support throughout the field work,[30, 68] and personal genuine interest and commitment for the research content on the part of the interviewers.[30, 77] Thus, cross-cultural comparability may be to an unknown degree hampered by the uneven degree of training, experience, and sophistication of employed interviewers and field workers.

Furthermore, we know very little about the nature of the effect of the interviewers' age, sex, social class, and attitudes about the studied subjects upon the nature of responses elicited. Some research on this area has shown that definite relationships exist between the interviewers' characteristics and the nature of obtained responses;[28, 35, 38, 75, 76, 84] the available knowledge, however, does not permit investigators in a given situation to control for these effects or to choose the kind of interviewers he ought to have. Although some investigators do select their interviewers at least in terms of social class, sex, and age, their attitudinal make-up is hardly ever controlled. Some exceptions to this are Grimshaw's and Safilios-Rothschild's research. In interviewing upper class Peruvian women, Grimshaw[33] had to use "elite" female strangers because male interviewers were not acceptable by husbands and upper class Peruvian women could not be persuaded to act as interviewers. Safilios-Rothschild[68] chose female interviewers from respective classes to interview a sample of Athenian women stratified for social class. Thus, although we know that this uncontrolled variability, especially in cross-cultural research, may in some way interfere with the comparability of

82

data, we cannot even estimate the degree or nature of incomparability that is introduced.

Strategies and Models of Cross-Cultural Research

The older model of cross-cultural research, according to which most social psychiatric data were collected in the past, was that of an American research team and less often a sole investigator going to another culture to replicate an earlier American study. Sometimes, this research team included some indigenous collaborators but this was not a rule. This team was often interdisciplinary, involving psychiatrists and anthropologists and less often sociologists. As such, it often generated well-known interprofessional conflicts, especially since social scientists always resented their subordination by the higher status-ranking and more highly paid psychiatrists. Because of the involvement of anthropologists on the team, cross-cultural research in this area was sometimes of the "safari" or the "parachute" type in which the investigators had minimal immersion in the studied culture and rather exploitative relationships with the scientists native to the area.

The reasons for the above type of a research model were: (1) the frequent lack of specialists-researchers in some of the chosen, theoretically-relevant developing societies; (2) the local unavailability of funds for research as well as of research time because of extremely heavy service loads for psychiatrists or the need to accept governmental social policy and development jobs for social scientists in most developing countries where research of any kind is considered a luxury item; and (3) the rather frequent lack of research training, experience, and sophistication on the part of interested indigenous psychiatrists and social scientists, precluding collaboration on an equal basis.

These limitations, however, do not hold true in a continuously increasing number of developing societies; consequently, new strategies of cross-cultural research are being developed. These strategies now actively involve scientists indigenous to the area on an equal basis. This involvement has come as a result of pressure since local institutions, administrators, and scientists were not willing to cooperate in any way unless they were included. This requirement of involvement has a double benefit for the studied society itself since these scientists acquire valuable research experience and knowledge from collaborating with others and the research findings will be also published in the local language so that they become available to local administrators, scientists, and students.

Several types of such collaboration have been suggested and tried out. Duijker and Stein[25] distinguish between successive and concurrent data gathering operations, that is, between repetitive and joint development of the research project. Only the latter type of research operation requires formal, preplanned cooperation between investigators in each country. They suggest a combination of these two types of collaboration by establishing an interdependent relationship between research initiators and data-gatherers through a rotation of roles between institutions in the different countries. Actually, up to now most of the comparative studies in any field have been of the successive data gathering type, investigators having become interested at different times in conducting similar studies in different countries. An example of such research on an extensive scale has been the series of studies on family structure modeled after Blood and Wolfe's Detroit Study and carried out with some modifications in Japan, Belgium, France, Greece, Spain and Yugoslavia. The original American study was done by Blood and Wolfe.[8] The replication studies were undertaken by: Blood;[7] De Bie and associates;[18] Michel;[50] Safilios-Rothschild;[66] and Buric and Zecevic.[9] The greatest shortcoming of this pattern of successive data gathering has been the lack of common organization and planning, resulting in poor comparability.

In some cases of small comparative studies, the same investigator replicated, with few modifications, the same study, usually in two societies; his native country and the one in which he was trained and/or had lived for a considerable number of years. The latter country was usually the United States; in a few cases, however, the investigators were Americans who had lived for several years in another country.

Scheuch[73] has emphasized the necessity of collaboration from the early stages of a research project. According to him, the phase during which a research concern is being translated into a tentative design is when closer collaboration and agreement than now exists is of utmost importance. Such a research strategy would prevent the imposing of a conceptual schema developed in one country on other countries where investigators have different conceptual orientations, and would eventually contribute to the formulation of international sociological theories.

Recently a cross-cultural family project undertaken by an international team of five researchers has come close to the joint development strategy of cross-cultural research.* First, a general conceptual framework was developed. Then, through a variety of consortium research meetings of interested investigators from different countries, the final form of the research design, methodology, and conceptualization to be used in the comparative research are jointly being decided. Most of the collaborating investigators indigenous to the country are highly qualified, have extensive research experience, and have been able to secure locally all or most of the necessary funds for the research. Everyone is not starting the research project in his country at the same time, but at each initiation all investigators participate in the decision-making process. Probably, this strategy of cross-cultural research in which each researcher, or team, from each country participates in all aspects of research planning and decision-making from a very early stage and on an equal basis with everyone will become the prevalent

---

*We are referring to the Cross-National Research Studies on the Family, organized by Marvin B. Sussman, Betty E. Cogswell, Constantina Safilios-Rothschild, Erwin K. Scheuch, and Robert Winch and funded by N.I.C.H.H.D.

type of strategy in the future. One distinct advantage of this research model is its solution to the problem of increasingly difficult funding of cross-cultural research through the financial resources of one country, namely the United States. By lending international standing and prestige to a particular research undertaking, governments, national and regional institutions, and foundations become interested and willing to provide the necessary funds to individual native researchers. The financial independence of each researcher enables him to be a full-fledged collaborator in an international research project. Furthermore, particularly in the case of research in psychiatric sociology, interdisciplinary teams of psychiatrists and social scientists function quite well in countries where psychiatrists have as low prestige and monetary rewards as social scientists and a good research relationship has already been established. Greece is an example of a country in which such interdisciplinary teams work quite smoothly and successfully.

The Language Barrier

The language barrier, as Osgood named it, is basic as well as inevitable in cross-cultural research. Many conceptual difficulties and incomparabilities originate from this basic issue. The translation of instruments, questions, and schedules is besieged by a variety of problems and ironically, a good, or faithful, translation does not necessarily represent a good adaptation.[58] Actually, as it has been argued by several cross-cultural investigators, it is more important that the translated units are equivalent rather than exactly the same; that is, the translation is such that conceptually equivalent questions are asked in each sociocultural setting so that there is some certainty that the obtained responses are comparable.[3]

Strategies for increasing linguistic equivalence of translation have been suggested by Osgood,[58] Prince and Mombour,[60] and Warner and Campbell.[82] All these suggested strategies are based upon variations of back translations and the use of accomplished bilingual individuals in order to validate the equivalence in both languages. Of course, the latter technique is of limited use in cross-cultural studies involving a number of societies and requiring equivalence of instruments used in all societies. Somewhat more sophisticated suggestions such as the "iterative approach" have been made by Anderson, and by Warner and Campbell. Anderson[3] suggests the use of alternate forms obtained from one or more back-translated versions. These alternate forms approach the measurement of the same conceptual realm with somewhat different linguistic irrelevancies. These forms may be used to generate added versions in each language through several iterations of the back-translation procedure. Although costly, the result permits randomization of the effects of language and translation through the use of multiple forms. Warner and Campbell,[82] on the other hand, suggest the use of multiple items and at least two items per concept, each pair sharing no key words but being as identical as possible in meaning. Then they suggest analyzing the results item by item rather than solely by total score; if factor analysis is involved, it should be carried out in both languages. In computing factor scores, only those items that show up on the same factors in all examined cultures should be used. However, as Scheuch[73] points out, even the most sophisticated translation strategies do not satisfactorily cope with the basic problem of conceptual equivalence for which no specific strategies or procedures have been formulated.

Although the use of verbal instruments encounters language barriers, the use of nonverbal tasks does not solve the problem of translation and equivalence, it just changes the nature of the problem.[3] Nonverbal procedures and instruments should be used in addition rather than instead of verbal instruments and should be based upon definite concepts and assumptions that require translation and adaptation for conceptual equivalence as much as verbal procedures.[82]

COLLECTING THE DATA: SURVEYS
VERSUS CRITICAL INTERVIEWS
AND INSTRUMENT CONSTRUCTION

The clinical interview has been the traditional technique of data collecting in social psychiatric research. Despite the difficulty of establishing the reliability or validity of the data thus collected, the results can be quite satisfactory when the interviewer is indigenous, has a good understanding of the culture, can establish good rapport with people, and conceptualizes some kind of standard questions. However, within the context of cross-cultural research, it is difficult to assume that investigators in several countries will conduct clinical interviews in a similar way so that the resulting data can be comparable. Therefore, some researchers even reject psychiatric diagnoses based solely on clinical information because of their lack of validity. Instead, they recommend a structured questionnaire that provides a standard, explicit set of data for psychiatric assessment.[24] This solution, however, also has some comparability problems.

There are two outstanding cases in which a symptom checklist developed and tested in one country was administered in another. The 22-symptom checklist developed in the Midtown Manhattan Study was administered to samples of women in Mexico City and Tehuantepee without any cultural adaptations. The investigator concluded that the data would have been much more meaningful had multiple scales covering different dimensions of mental disorder (anxiety, depression, suspiciousness, rigidity, etc.) been carefully pretested in several cultures in order "to achieve some comparability of meaning."[40] While this procedure has never been followed exactly, Murphy and Hughes[54] examined the possibility of using the Health Opinion Survey, a list of psychophysiological symptoms selected and standardized by Macmillan in the Stirling County Study, in an Eskimo population. They found that four out of the twenty questions were inappropriate for the Eskimo population because they referred to states of being that were usually experienced by all of them at least "sometimes;"[54] however, the majority of items seemed to be useful indicators. Although the symptom checklist could be modified to become more sensitive for the Eskimo culture, it was judged to be generally valid since it could spot illness among the Eskimos, but was not effective in distinguishing "wellness."[54]

The problem of cross-cultural equivalence and comparability is a general methodological problem common to all questionnaires or scales measuring the "same" concept(s) in a number of different sociocultural settings. Two different types of methodological procedures have been suggested in order to maximize comparability of instruments. One is essentially as follows: a large list of questions covering a full spectrum; for example significant symptoms of psychiatric disorders, should be administered to different cultural settings. Only those items that distinguish the mentally ill from the well in each culture would be selected and combined into a "core set of universally appropriate questions."[54] Although this recommendation sounds ideal, it has several practical and methodological shortcomings, such as requiring long and expensive pretesting of procedures for reliable identification of psychiatric cases and possible bias from having omitted significant and discriminating culture-specific questions about psychiatric disorders. Thus, although exactly the same questions are being asked in all studied cultures, the degree of comparability is not perfect.

For this reason, a second methodological recommendation aims at arriving not at an identical set of questions but rather at "equivalent" sets of indicators, some of which may be identical in all cultures and some culture-specific but highly intercorrelated with the identical ones. It has been demonstrated that the inclusion of nation-specific items tends to increase the reliability of the scale.[58, 61] This technique can also solve the difficult problem involved in the cross-cultural study of concepts that are unidimensional in one culture and multidimensional in another, or of concepts, such as alienation, that require a completely different set of indicators or different measurement techniques in different cultures.[34, 58] The second recommendation is more promising because of the degree of flexibility that it provides, the assurance of conceptual equivalence, and the wide applicability it has to all kinds of concepts and all types of cultural settings.

The following are some examples of cross-cultural differential perception, occurring with the use of objective instruments. When Taylor's Manifest Anxiety Scale was administered in Japan, a number of problems were encountered; some items were not definite enough and the Japanese subjects found it difficult to answer the many negatively phrased expressions. After the appropriate revisions, however, the degree of reliability was found to be satisfactory.[57] Similarly, Biesheuvel[6] mentions the relative clumsiness of African respondents when presented with a test requiring manipulative skills, such as the Wechsler performance scale. This is especially apparent in children who have not had much opportunity to play with blocks or puzzles.

African Blacks' difficulties in dealing with three-dimensional perception of two-dimensional pictures have been noted, among others, by Deregowski[21] and by Dawson.[17] Dawson has pointed out that such difficulties often interfere with performance on the block-design subtest of the Wechsler Scale. There is some evidence that this deficiency is caused by physiological as well as psychological factors and is accompanied by strong field dependence.[17]

Projective techniques, although nonverbal, also need modifications for use successfully in other cultures. Because the content of pictures or even of the white empty space in Rorschach cards,[1] may have entirely different connotations, their validity must be separately established for each country.[42] For example, the original Murray TAT cards could not be used in India because the social situations it portrayed did not have counterparts in India; it could be used, however, after a new series of pictures was developed that represented Indian counterparts of similar social situations.[13]

Comparability of Data: The Crux of the Matter

If cross-cultural research in any area of inquiry is to fulfill its promise of helping establish universal laws and of "catching strategic variables in new ranges,"[22] comparability of the gathered data must be assured. The basic question is: "When is the same really the same?"[51] As we saw in the previous section, some feel that comparability is best safeguarded through "phenomenal identity" and others through "conceptual" or "functional" equivalence as defended by Osgood[58] and Scheuch.[73] The issue arises in all research procedures, in sampling, design, and construction of instruments as well as in the basic conceptualization and definitions of independent and dependent variables.[81] The research question itself must be appropriately conceptualized; despite efforts to establish "universal categories," not all research problems can be investigated in all societies. As Lesser and Kandel[41] have pointed out, measurement in cross-cultural research must assess variables that: (1) exist in each society, (2) are expressed in each society and (3) are elicited by stimuli equivalent in meaning in each society. Unless these precautions are taken, one may be measuring nonexistent opinions in some cultures by asking questions about entities that do not exist.[51, 59] For example, Whyte and Williams[83] found that Peruvian blue collar workers were not accustomed to thinking about their relationships with the supervisors in as many dimensions as were American workers. Scheuch[73] even questions the widely accepted assumption of considering each respondent as a unit carrying opinions and attributes; he observes that individuals in certain cultures may not be willing or at liberty to voice an opinion.

There are also a number of extraneous variables that are very difficult to control but that may more or less interfere with the degree of comparability of findings: test-taking or interview familiarity; importance of status, age, sex, or attitudinal differences between interviewer and respondent; effect of social desirability framework; and "courtesy bias" (that is, the tendency of the respondent to try to please the interviewer).[41] The effect of each of these factors may take divergent directions in different cultures. For example, the courtesy bias in Japan may be responsible for an underestimation of the respondent's achievement while in the Middle East, the same bias would tend to produce an overestimation of the respondent's achievement.[51] In order to be able to correct the findings influenced by such biases, supplementary studies of their effects in different cultures are necessary.

SPECIFIC METHODOLOGICAL PROBLEMS OF CROSS-CULTURAL RESEARCH IN PSYCHIATRIC SOCIOLOGY

Sampling Problems

Sampling problems are generic to all cross-cultural research and some are more specific to social psychiatric research. Universal problems involve the appropriateness and feasibility of samples of societies as well as the respondent samples within each culture. For example, one issue revolves around the appropriateness and feasibility of random, representative samples versus "scope" samples which can be of great value in research of an analytical nature. While the nature of the research usually spells out rather clearly the sampling requirements, both representativeness within a society and comparability among societies are required.[73, 58] Therefore, in order to establish both simultaneously, the researcher is often forced to make compromises and to occasionally sacrifice rigorousness and precision.[41]

Another issue revolves around identical sampling versus culturally equivalent sampling procedures. Scheuch draws our attention to the fact that identical sampling procedures may not only be insufficient in achieving comparability, but may even be harmful because significant aspects of the universe to be studied are not sampled. For example, Christensen[14] mentions that college student samples in Denmark and the United States are not comparable because of different selective proportions of the population that attend a university in the two countries.

The sampling of societies to be included in a particular cross-cultural research study is also problematic. Usually, only two cultures have been compared, one of them being the United States since cross-cultural research is typically undertaken by an American investigator on an exchange program in another country or by a foreign scholar who was trained in the United States and became interested in conducting comparative research. Even when a number of cultures are involved, the determining factors most often have been accidental or purely practical such as, the investigator's acquaintance with researchers in other countries who are willing to collaborate. Ideally, of course, societies should be chosen according to a conceptual criterion; the known or theoretically expected degree of variation on a crucial variable under study or the location of a society in a cell of a pertinent societal typology. The former type of criterion requires a very good knowledge of the society under consideration while the latter requires a societal typology that permits the clear-cut classification of all societies and the inclusion of basic variables that render it relevant for a variety of research projects.

Most of the existing typologies classify societies according to their degree of industrial and economic development. Sawyer,[72] for instance, classifies nations according to political system, size, and wealth. Another interesting societal typology is that developed by Dechmann and associates,[19] classifying nations mainly by the opportunities for upward mobility that they offer their inhabitants. Nations are categorized by four dimensions: interest articulation by associational groups, interest by institutional groups, ascriptiveness of the political elite, and cultural (linguistic) heterogeneity. Combinations of varying degrees of these four variables give rise to the definition of four broad descriptive types: the Traditional Feudal Society, the Modernizing Sectionalist Society, the Mobilization System Society, and the Modern Industrial Society. These four types are assumed to define a developmental sequence from a traditional to a modern society. Nations categorized at the lower end of the sequence are characterized by extreme dependency, a high power deficit, and a very low degree of development. Those at the upper end are characterized by high independence, a high power excess, and the highest degree of development. For further refinement of the typology, two additional dimensions of power, ascribed and achieved, are also introduced. A number of structural variables are then used to quantitatively describe the four types of nations. The main variables are level of education, percentage of towns with a population over 100,000, Gross National Product, level of income per capita, and of divisions labor. Data presented for 1950, 1955, and 1960 show, on the whole, that the postulated developmental sequence is well reflected in these quantitative measures.[19] Such a typology could be extremely useful in a cross-cultural project, allowing for the equating of a number of cultures on certain dimensions, while others would be purposefully varied.

Besides the sampling of entire cultures, another methodological issue is whether one should consider an entire country as a unit, thus ignoring deviations from an overall national representation, or should instead take advantage of intranational differences. As Linz and de Miquel[43] showed, Spain is made up of "eight Spains," each differing with regard to level of economic development; social structure; level of education; linguistic, cultural, and political tradition; religious climate; social mobilization; values, norms, basic personality, and family patterns. The same intranational variance holds true in Yugoslavia and India. Once the different areas and communities could be carefully delineated according to different structural and modernization variables. As has been done with Finnish communities,[62] the comparability of cross-cultural data could be maximized by collecting data in the same type of community in each culture. For example, one could compare family members' degree of tolerance toward mental illness in traditional, transitional, or modern urban communities in different cultures instead of comparing whole cultures or accidentally selected cities in each culture.

Social psychiatric research also encounters specific sampling problems which merit special attention. Census or other official statistics are often of little use even when they are readily available, although few countries have well organized

90

records of hospitalized mental patients. When such statistics are available, however, they usually include those hospitalized in public hospitals and only some of those in private hospitals. In developing countries, the private psychiatric clinics are very often the small business undertakings of one or two psychiatrists who, because of tax purposes, do not report the exact number of patients. Furthermore, upper and upper-middle class patients in all societies tend to be hospitalized much less frequently than those in lower classes, this holding true for the first as well as for subsequent periods of hospitalization. This often is due to a greater reluctance on the part of psychiatrists to hospitalize an important person, coping instead with his problems in the office setting. In the case of hospitalization, patients who are financially well-off fare better, probably because of their families' greater range of resources available for care and supervision.[55] In an epidemiological study where an effort was made to locate private outpatients, the success rate was mediocre because a number of psychiatrists were unwilling to report the exact number of cases they were treating. In some developing countries, there are no exclusive private psychiatric clinics and the degree of social stigma attached, especially to hospitalization for mental illness, is very potent. Consequently, many patients in the upper classes go abroad when they are in need of long-term psychiatric treatment and hospitalization. For example, Greek upper and upper-middle class patients go to psychiatric clinics in Switzerland or France, while middle class patients go to Austrian clinics which are financially more accessible to middle income persons.[64] It seems obvious, therefore, that there is a serious degree of underestimation concerning the numbers of persons, particularly those from the middle and upper classes, who are, or have been, under psychiatric treatment.

Epidemiological studies, in addition to their great cost, experience a tremendous number of difficulties even when they are restricted to a particular urban setting. When they are conducted on a nationwide basis, the problems are multiplied. In many developing countries the degree of administrative and staff cooperation with research studies, as well as the availability of interviewing or survey personnel, diminishes linearly with the distance from the capital. Even when epidemiological studies of the prevalence of mental illness are successfully carried out on a nationwide basis, serious methodological questions remain about the validity of the data if they are covering only hospitalized rates. The latter tend to reflect much more the adequacy of available facilities and the tendency to seek hospitalization rather than the need for hospitalization.[5, 85, 24]

Even when an outpatient population has been adequately covered, the resulting prevalence rates are underestimates since in most societies there are at least as many people, if not more, who are mentally ill but are not being treated.[44] Some additional factors that may bias an incidence study, especially in primitive societies, are pointed out by Hunt.[37] Severe disturbances may be rare due to the low survival rate of dangerous psychotics in such societies. Neurotics, on the other hand, may not even be recognized as "mental cases" because they often get along fairly well in that kind of social milieu.

A combination of epidemiological studies covering both hospitalized patients and out-patients with interview studies of random samples of general populations would constitute the perfect solution. However, in societies where people are extremely sensitive about and reluctant to discuss their experiences with any kind of deviant or abnormal symptoms, the administration of symptoms lists (such as the one used in the Midtown Manhattan Study) may be met with a high refusal rate or with socially desirable responses.

In developing societies where the stigma attached to mental illness is extremely potent and carries severe sanctions pervading all life sectors of the mentally ill and all their close relatives, there is usually considerable tolerance of a wide range of symptomatology as well as a considerable unwillingness to assume the mentally disturbed role, or to define someone else as being mentally ill. Because of this, the early stages of mental disturbance, definitional problems, and mechanisms of coping with mental disturbance can only be studied *retrospectively*. It is not possible to study anything more than definitions of mental illness, attitudes toward psychiatrists, mental illness, and hospitalization and coping mechanisms dealing with hypothetical mental disturbances on samples of general populations. Questions about the presence of mental illness or its symptomatology do not give reliable information because there is a considerable degree of refusal and understatement concerning such disclosure.

In conclusion, because patients in the middle and upper classes are seldom available in most cross-cultural social psychiatric research—with the exception of attitudinal research—most formulated hypotheses and conclusions have been based upon predominantly lower-working and lower-middle class populations of hospitalized patients or outpatients. In the study by Angrist and associates,[32] 84 per cent of the women patients belonged to the lower or lower-middle class. Such significant sampling restrictions have been true for such work as that by Yarrow and associates,[86] Clausen and Yarrow,[15] and Schwartz[74] and the replications of these studies in Greece by Safilios-Rothschild[67] as well as Rogler and Hollingshead's[63] and Bell and Zucker's[4] studies.

The Ethics of Cross-Cultural Psychiatric Research

Ethical problems universal in cross-cultural research include the invasion of privacy and the questions of disguise of purpose and anonymity. In cross-cultural psychiatric research, however, some of these ethical problems are even more serious and in some cases, no research can be carried out unless some of these principles are partially compromised. For example, due to the social stigma attached to mental illness in most developing societies, the relatives of a mentally ill person may not agree to talk with anyone but the treating psychiatrists. Thus, a sociologist who wishes to carry out research on the meaning of mental illness in the family or on the labeling stages of mental illness must be presented under the disguise of a psychiatrist (wearing the white coat and all) in order to secure interviews with the patients relatives. While it is true that the extensive family data that the research sociologist gathers may be also helpful to the treating psychiatrist, the psychiatrist may not always be interested, have faith in or have access to such information. The ethical dilemma remains: does the sociologist have the right to secure the respondents' cooperation and to gather intimate data under false pretenses even when such pretenses are scientific and not manipulative?

THE MEASUREMENT AND COMPARABILITY OF SOCIAL CLASS AND SOCIAL MOBILITY ACROSS NATIONS

In most comparative studies in psychiatric sociology social class is a central variable. Despite its central place in most areas of sociological research and despite much specific research on the measurement of social class, few of the methodological problems have been successfully solved. Indeed, because of the numerous problems, cross-cultural comparisons of social class-related variables have become extremely difficult and of doubtful validity.

Some of the outstanding methodological problems involved in the measurement of social class are:

(1) Until recently social class has usually been calculated on the basis of the education and occupation of an adult male. Thus, the social class of married women has always been calculated on the basis of her husband's education and occupation. Likewise, the social class of a teenager or young adult has been calculated on the basis of his father's education and occupation. While this operation may have never been accurate, it is increasingly becoming erroneous and misleading. Haug and Sussman[36] found in a recent national survey sample that in 31.9 per cent of the cases the wife's occupational level was higher than that of her husband and that in 24.3 per cent of the cases the wife's educational level was higher than that of her husband. They found that the largest differences occur among husbands who are manual workers or who had not finished high school. We cannot assume that the wife's higher occupational and/or educational level have no influence upon the family's social class standing. This omission of the wife's contribution to the social class standing is particularly important when the subjects under study are women and are accordingly over- or underestimated. The magnitude of the problem is particularly apparent since in other societies, equally or less developed than the United States, a greater percentage of women work in highly prestigious and skilled occupations.[70] Even in those developing societies in which few women work, increasingly more of them are achieving a higher level of education than men. Because of this inaccuracy, some investigators tend to rely more heavily on education than on social class since it is a much more sensitive variable for distinguishing between groups of women, or groups of men, with respect to their values and attitudes, especially those reflecting social, familial, or individual modernity. Sociological research indicates that education differentiates between men and women with regard to family size, attitudes toward women's employment, definitions of marital roles, attitudes toward psychiatrists and mental illness, and familial power struc-

ture.[16, 23, 66, 69, 77] A degree of inaccuracy is also present when the social class of teenagers and young adults is measured on the basis of their fathers' education and occupation. It is becoming increasingly common in all societies for children to achieve a higher level of education than their parents, and thereby the potential for a higher occupational level.

(2) In many societies, especially those that are developing, (for example, Greece) the social class standing of the family is frequently greatly influenced, if not determined, by the wife's personal property. Thus, although the wife may not work and her educational level may be lower than that of her husband, she may in fact determine the social class standing of the family because the revenues from her property permit them to live at a level above that accorded to the husband's social class position. This does not occur only in the case of very rich women; it happens as well with average or even with low income families. In the latter case, a small additional revenue may adjust the family's financial status just enough to keep them above the poverty level. Traditional social class techniques of measurement are completely insensitive to these very important social class determinants.

(3) In most societies there are no standardized and validated occupational rankings that would permit an investigator to rank occupations according to their social prestige. It is interesting to note studies that show similar prestige ranking of occupations in a variety of countries such as, Japan, Great Britain, the United States, Germany, and Indonesia.[10, 39] These results were replicated by Svalastoga[79] when Scandinavia was compared to the above countries. This striking similarity may, however, be only artificial because the few occupations that were studied are well-known and highly prestigious professions which have a much greater probability to receive a similar ranking. However, in social psychiatric studies in which the usual sample is made up of people in lower-middle and lower class occupations, many of which are not usually included in the ranked lists of occupations, the estimated rankings assigned to these occupations are often arbitrary and of very questionable validity. Furthermore, since there is evidence that the higher an occupation is evaluated, the greater the consensus of difference regarding its ranking,[39, 52] it can be expected that there is a high degree of dispersion of opinions about the occupations usually represented in social psychiatric research studies.

It is necessary to also consider that very rarely has one of the American social class measures (for example, Hollingshead's Two Factor Index of Social Position) been validated in another country; therefore, it is quite erroneous to assume that it is valid without some modification, especially for developing societies. For example, Hollingshead's lower weighting of education may be erroneous for many developing societies in which education may carry the same weight as occupation. Substantiation for this fact was found in Greece.[65]

Due to the lack of validated measurements of social class in most other societies, investigators often attempt to improvise. These improvisations render cross-cultural, comparative data by social class rather doubtful and unreliable.

Until some of the previously described methodological problems are solved, level of education alone could be used as an instrument of measurement. Again there are serious problems of comparison here because the same level of education has a completely different type of effect upon one's values and attitudes according to the particular societal level of development. However, once the level of education that differentiates between men and women of opposing views (the critical level of education being different for men and women) is known, it is possible to take this into consideration in comparing subjects in different societies with respect to attitudes toward psychiatrists, mental hospitals, and hospitalization.

(4)   Social psychiatric studies have seldom considered the subjective, as well as objective measure of social class. Evidence from available research studies points, however, to considerable discrepancies between what the investigator assigned as an individual's social class on the basis of his education and occupation and the social class that the respondent assigned to himself.[11, 12, 47, 65] In addition, there are definite patterns that individuals follow in over- or underestimating their social class standing.

When a researcher is interested in investigating the incidence of psychiatric disorders, the labeling of such disorders, or attitudes toward mental illness and psychiatrists, he might find that a person's subjective social class standing, or the nature of the discrepancy between this subjective assignment and a more objective one, may be a much more sensitive variable than the objective measurement of social class *per se*. These additional dimensions of social class may have a considerble explanatory power with respect to many of the phenomena of central interest to psychiatric sociologists and may help refine the nature of existing relationships because they tend to indicate more directly the respondents' real values and needs. For example, it may be that in certain types of societies, those who aspire to middle class status while they are lower class according to objective criteria, show a higher incidence of schizophrenia than those of subjective and objective middle class standing.

(5)   Cross-cultural comparisons very seldom take into consideration the various type of social differentiation in, and the distribution of the population in the social classes. Thus, they ignore the fact that in some of the little-urbanized developing societies, the largest segment of the population is lower class, only a small segment being middle or upper class. In other highly urbanized but not highly industrialized developing countries, there may be a sizeable middle class.

The significant question is: What is the meaning and the consequences of the differential distribution of population in each social class in various types of societies? There is some evidence that the size of the lower class in a society, usually correlated with the extent of potential upward social mobility, determines the nature of the cultural stereotypes and images attached to lower class people. Assuming that some degree of upward mobility is possible, the larger the social class in a society, the smaller the possibility of mobility, the more the poor, and the lower class people are seen as honest, hard-working reliable, good people who have remained poor because of their integrity and high moral standards. In such societies, the image of the rich is quite negative and includes such traits as ruthlessness, cruelty, compromise of moral and humanitarian principles, and unhappiness. On the contrary, in societies in which the lower class is not sizeable and there is a considerable degree of upward social mobility based upon ability or education, the cultural stereotypes are completely different. The poor are portrayed as lazy, passive, and immoral individuals whose status is entirely "their own fault." Those more financially well-off are viewed as meriting, hardworking, and admirable, but not necessarily very honest.[65]

The degree of class consciousness may be greatly influenced by the size of a class and the cultural stereotypes attached to it. Thus, it may be that the level of class consciousness is much higher when its size is quite large and positive stereotypes are attached to it that encourage people to identify with it.

(6) The inherent unreliability of diagnostic procedures may systematically bias the data generated with regard to the respondents' social status. As Hunt[37] points out, when the diagnosis for an individual is uncertain, a schizophrenic diagnosis is in some measure a function of his social status.

These factors ought to be taken into consideration in the construction of a societal typology that would render cross-cultural comparisons of phenomena in correlation with social class more meaningful and amenable to the formulation of valid social theory.

In addition to social class, social mobility has also been frequently studied with respect to the incidence of mental disorders. Measuring the variable of social mobility in any particular society, may cause serious methodological problems when cross-cultural comparisons are attempted.

First, the degree of a respondent's social mobility is either measured in comparison to a previous point in his own career (such as first occupation or occupation 5 or 10 years ago) or in comparison to his father's occupation. In studying the latter type of intergenerational mobility, the father's usual or last main occupation is most often used as a point of comparison. This occupational index, however, may not be very valid if the father's occupational career was not stable but included periods of upward or downward social mobility and/or significant changes of occupation. Furthermore, the validity of these comparisons may be compromised because drastic social changes may have significantly altered the prestige of some occupations from the father's to the son's generation. Although it appears that some mobility has occurred, in actual fact, there has been no change. In many societies, even when the son is in his late 20's or early 30's, it is still early to evaluate the level of occupational standing that he will eventually reach and measurement at this point may seriously underestimate his status. Finally, even when the same degree of inter- or intragenerational mobility is found in different societies, it is not necessarily the same phenomenon with the same consequences, especially for mental health. Depending upon the facility with which one can become upwardly mobile, the prevalence and social acceptance of such people, and the nature of the means one has to use in order to achieve upward mobility, the mobility phenomenon varies significantly. These typological variations are seldom taken into consideration in the study of the relationship between social mobility and mental illness.[79]

Second, in measuring social mobility in developing countries, whether intra- or intergenerationally, one is met with the frequent problem of evaluating the rural or urban transition that constitutes change to an urban occupation.[9] Besides the difficulty of evaluating the degree of mobility involved in the transition from a rural to an urban occupation, the intervening variable of migration may play an important role in the relationships studied in social psychiatric research, especially in the case of recent migration. (For further information see, "Methodological Problems in Studying the Relationship between Migration and Mental Illness."). This problem is particularly frequent when one studies intergenerational mobility or when the sampled population consists of mainly the urban lower class, which is of recent rural origin in most developing countries. Since the lower class is the usual population sampled in social psychiatric studies, this situation is particularly relevant. There is really no objective or accurate technique for determining the degree of social mobility entailed in the rural-to-urban occupational transition and, therefore, the degree of social mobility assigned varies from researcher to researcher and from society to society.

Third, when cross-cultural comparisons of social mobility from one type of occupational category to another are attempted, the groupings of the occupations become broad in order to allow such comparisons. Consequently very little of the actual social mobility is accounted for and the resulting comparisons are of doubtful validity. Fox and Miller[29] have pointed out that mobility typically measured in terms of "manual and nonmanual" categories is grossly inadequate because it neglects the intrastratum progress which in many countries is the most prevalent type.

Methodological Problems in Studying the Relationship Between Migration and Mental Illness

We shall deal here only with immigration in relation to mental illness. Emigration may be voluntary or forced with regard to idiosyncratic motives regardless of the official classification that may be given to an immigrant's move. For example, it has been found that some of the Hungarian refugees of 1956 left their country for nonpolitical reasons and were, in fact, voluntary migrants.[49] The consequences of each type of emigration are very different for one's social adaptation and mental health status. Despite this, this typological distinction has seldom been taken into consideration in epidemiological studies of hospitalization for mental illness among immigrants.

The main methodological problem involved in investigations of the relationship between immigration and mental illness, however, is the fact that the epidemiological data based upon immigrants must be compared to other similar data before they can become meaningful. The basis for comparison has usually been the hospitalization rates of the native population without any standardization for age, sex and, social class—characteristics usually distributed differently among immigrants than among natives and varying considerably with each immigrant group or immigration periods.[48] Furthermore, the natives are very often intracultural migrants; the effects of such migration are not to be neglected since it also may contribute to the overall mental health status of the population. For example, in one study it was found that, with respect to mental health status, immigrants were intermediary between native New Yorkers and out-of-state migrants.[45] Hospitalization rates for immigrants have seldom been compared to those in their native country, whenever such a comparison was made, however, the rates had not been standardized, so the two sets of data were not comparable. Thus, it is quite possible that in many cases, the greater incidence of mental illness found among immigrants than among natives could be attributed to the differential distribution of the two groups along the social class continuum or to the change in degree of social mobility from their country of origin.

Two further methodological shortcomings of most migration studies are:[48] (1) overlooking the immigrants' length of stay in the new land and (2) the diagnostic artifacts involved in the labeling of behavioral acts representing normal behavior within another cultural setting, especially during the stressful acculturation process, as symptoms indicating mental illness and requiring hospitalization. The omission of the variable of length-of-stay is significant because there is considerable evidence that the incidence of mental illness among immigrants is very high during the first year and declines rapidly thereafter.[26, 46] The first year is the time during which the immigrant must cope with cultural shock and make major adjustments. The stress of this adaptation often being so overwhelming that symptomatology indicative of mental illness may be an understandable situation reaction.

It would be extremely fruitful to undertake cross-cultural studies of the relationship between immigration and mental illness in countries that attract people from the same cultures but that have very different immigration laws and assimilation models such as, the United States, Canada, New Zealand, Australia, Brazil, Argentina, Great Britain, and Germany.

The Cross-Cultural Study of Psychiatric Disorders: Diagnostic Problems

In an earlier section we examined the sampling problems that besiege epidemiological as well as other types of social psychiatric studies. Let us turn to another serious and basic problem, the diagnoses of psychiatric disorders given by psychiatrists in different countries.

First, the comparability of diagnoses made by psychiatrists in different cultures is greatly hampered by the lack of unanimity of opinion regarding psychiatric diagnostic terminology as well as by the presence of symptoms necessary to assign a patient to a particular diagnostic category.[31, 24, 56] The quality and type of training of psychiatrists varies greatly not only with the country but also with the physician.[53, 85] The degree of variation in the psychiatric training is particularly great in developing countries where psychiatrists have studied in different countries and are influenced by a variety of schools of thought. Thus, in Greece, one finds that psychiatrists have been trained in the United States, Britain, France, Germany, Austria, Italy, or less frequently in the Soviet Union. The clinical concepts, criteria, and diagnostic labels they use vary, not only according with the country but also according to the university or hospital in which they were trained.[20, 64, 80] Finally, when a research psychiatrist makes a diagnosis in a culture other than his own, he might be influenced by his own attitude toward not only the patient but also toward the entire culture, his interpreters, and his anthropologist colleagues.[71] Even indigenous psychiatrists cannot be expected to escape prevailing cultural values and beliefs and their diagnoses seem to be significantly influenced by them. For example, it was found that Mexican psychiatrists tend to view symptoms with a lesser degree of seriousness, particularly with regard to their female patients, than do their American counterparts.[27]

Second, the meaning of at least some behavioral acts and symptoms varies considerably from culture to culture. Psychiatrists must evaluate the observed or reported patterns of behavior and feeling in relation to prevailing cultural norms of behavior.[53, 71, 85] Since mental illness, like most types of deviance, necessitates a societal definition, a behavior which is defined as being abnormal in one social and cultural setting may be ignored, tolerated, accepted as normal or even venerated in other settings.[71] Numerous such examples can be found in the available psychiatric, anthropological, and social psychiatric literature.[67, 71, 85] As a result of the sociocultural variations in the definition of behavioral acts and because Western standards have often been viewed as the "ideal" according to which non-Western behavior and psychological makeup has been psychiatrically evaluated (especially by Western psychiatrists), some of the differences in diagnostic distributions are artifacts. On the other hand, it is entirely possible that psychiatrists from other countries may not diagnose mild cases of mental disorder because the presenting symptoms are not too dissimilar from the typical normal behavior in the physician's particular cultural milieu. For example, when paranoid thoughts, especially about intrigues involving one's work, are quite widespread in a culture, as is true in Greece, cases in which the beginning symptoms of schizophrenia are expressed in terms of such paranoid thoughts may be at first accepted as normal.[67] These definitional problems involved in diagnosis are generally much less misleading to indigenous psychiatrists than to foreign ones, but even so may interfere in the degree of comparability of rates of prevalence of psychiatric disorders in different countries.

Third, psychiatric disorders may, because of differences in social, cultural, nutritional or other factors, appear under different sets of symptoms in various societies. For example, those with schizophrenic disorders in East Asia, who are not Christian or Muslim very seldom have delusions of destruction and religious delusions. On the contrary, delusions of jealousy are much more frequently reported for Asian samples than for Euro-Americans and catatonic signs appear much more frequently among East Indians, American Indians and Mestizos than among other groups. Inappropriateness of affect, feelings of depersonalization, and hypochondriacal ideas were reported as infrequent symptoms in a large number of cultures.[53] However, a recent survey of 40 psychiatrists working in 27 countries showed that four out of twenty-six signs and symptoms of schizophrenia were frequent everywhere and, therefore, constitute the minimal criteria for diagnosis and represent a core for comparison. In a seminar on cross-cultural psychiatric diagnoses, anthropologists and psychiatrists drew the conclusion that syndromes, on the whole, were much more manageable than individual symptoms but that the complete diagnosis remained a challenge.[71]

To summarize, then, cross-cultural research in psychiatric sociology will markedly improve when the research sociologists and psychiatrists are able to clearly define and subsequently operationalize all dimensions involved in each concept used; and when the general methodological problems of cross-cultural research are successfully solved, hopefully through a truly collaborative and international research model.

REFERENCES

1. ABEL, T. M., AND HSU, F. L. K.: "Some Aspects of Personality of Chinese as Revealed by the Rorschach Test." *Rorschach Research Exchange* 13:285-301, 1949.
2. ANGRIST, S. A., LEFTON, M., DINITZ, S., AND PASAMANICK, B.: *Women After Treatment*. New York: Appleton-Century-Crofts, 1968. pp. 76-77.
3. ANDERSON, R. B. W.: "On the Comparability of Meaningful Stimuli in Cross-cultural Research." *Sociometry* 30:124-136, 1967.
4. BELL, N. W., AND ZUCKER, R. A.: "Family-hospital Relationships in a State Hospital Setting." *The International Journal of Social Psychiatry* 15:73-80, 1968.
5. BERNE, E.: "Difficulties of Comparative Psychiatry: The Fiji Islands." *The American Journal of Psychiatry* 116:104-109, 1959.
6. BIESHEUVEL, S.: "Psychological Tests and their Application to Non-European Peoples," in D. R. Price-Williams (ed.): *Cross-Cultural Studies*. England: Penguin Books, 1969, pp. 57-75.
7. BLOOD, R. O.: *Love Match and Arranged Marriages*. New York: The Free Press, 1967.
8. BLOOD, R. O., AND WOLFE, D. M. *Husbands and Wives*. New York: The Free Press, 1960.
9. BURIC, O., AND ZECEVIC, A.: "Family Authority, Marital Satisfaction, and the Social Network in Yugoslavia." *Journal of Marriage and the Family* 29:325-336, 1967.
10. CARTER, R. E., AND SEPULVEDA, O.: "Occupational Prestige in Santiago de Chile." *American Behavioral Scientist* 8:20-24, 1964.
11. CENTERS, R.: "The People of the U.S.A.—'a Self-Portrait'." *Fortune* 21:14, 1940.
12. CENTERS, R.: *The Psychology of Social Classes*. Princeton, N. J.: Princeton University Press, 1949.
13. CHOWDBURY, U.: "An Indian Modification of the Thematic Apperception Test." *Journal of Social Psychology* 51:245-263, 1960.
14. CHRISTENSEN, H. T.: "A Cross-cultural Comparison of Attitudes Toward Marital Infidelity." *International Journal of Comparative Sociology* 3:124-137, 1962.
15. CLAUSEN, J. A., AND YARROW, M. R.: "The Impact of Mental Illness and the Family." *Journal of Social Issues* 11:3-5, 1955.
16. DANDEKAR, K.: "Effect of Education on Fertility." World Population Conference, 1965, vol. 4, New York: United Nations. p. 148.
17. DAWSON, J. L. M.: "Cultural and Physiological Influences Upon Spatial-perceptual Processes in West-Africa, Part I." *International Journal of Psychology* 2:115-128, 1967.

18. DE BIE, P., et al.: *La Dyade Conjugale*. Bruxelles: Editions Vie Duvriere, 1968.
19. DECHMANN, M., BORNSHIER, V., ALBERTINI, B. V., BOSSHARDT, W., AND STUTZ, F. B.: A Typology of Nations. Zurich, Switzerland: *Bulletin of the Soziologisches Institut der Universitat Zurich*, 1967.
20. DEMERATH, N. J.: "Schizophrenia Among Primitives: The Present Status of Sociological Research." *American Journal of Psychiatry* 98:703-707, 1942.
21. DEREGOWSKI, J. B.: "Difficulties in Pictorial Depth Perception in Africa." *British Journal of Psychology* 59:195-204, 1968.
22. DEVEREUX, E. C., BRONFENBRENNER, U., AND SUCI, G. H.: "Patterns of Parent Behavior in the United States of America and the Federal Republic of Germany: A Cross-national Comparison." *International Social Science Journal* 14:488-506, 1962.
23. DINKEL, R. M.: Education and Fertility in the United States. Paper presented at the United Nations World Population Conference, Belgrade, Yugoslavia, 1965.
24. DOHRENWEND, B. P., AND DOHRENWEND, B. S.: "The Problem of Validity in Field Studies of Psychological Disorder." *Journal of Abnormal Psychology* 70 (February):52-69, 1965.
25. DUIJKER, H., AND STEIN, R.: "Organizational Aspects of Cross-National Social Research." Journal of Social Issues 10:8-24, 1954.
26. EITINGER, L.: Psykiatriske Undersokelser Blant Flyktninger I Norge. Oslo: Universitetsforlaget, 1958.
27. FABREGA, H. JR., AND WALLACE, C. A.: "How Physicians Judge Psychophysiologic Symptoms: A Cross-cultural study." *Transcultural Psychiatric Research* 5:173-174, 1968.
28. FELDMAN, J. J., HYMAN, H., AND HART, C. W.: "A Field Study of Interviewer Effects on the Quality of Survey Data." *Public Opinion Quarterly* 15:734-761, 1951.
29. FOX, T., AND MILLER, S. M.: "Intra-country Variations: Occupational Stratification and Mobility," in R. Bendix and S. M. Lipset (eds.): *Class, Status, and Power,* 2nd edition. New York: The Free Press, 1966, pp. 574-581.
30. FREY, F. W.: "Surveying Peasant Attitudes in Turkey." *Public Opinion Quarterly* 27:335-355, 1963.
31. GAITONDE, M. R.: "Cross-cultural Study of the Psychiatric Syndromes in Out-patient Clinics in Bombay, India and Topeka, Kansas." *International Journal of Social Psychiatry* 4:98-104, 1958.
32. GLASS, D. V. (ed.): *Social Mobility in Britain.* London: Routledge and Kegan Paul, Ltd., 1954.
33. GRIMSHAW, A. D.: Accessibility of Elites. Unpublished paper, 1969.
34. HALLER, A. O.: Some Unknowns in the Relation of Behavior Changes to Value Changes. University of Wisconsin. Unpublished paper, 1965.
35. HANSON, R. H., AND MARKS, E. S.: "Influence of the Interviewer on the Accuracy of Survey Results." *Journal of American Statistical Association* 53:635-655, 1958.
36. HAUG, M. R., AND SUSSMAN, M. B.: Social Class Measurement: Some Problems and Proposals. Paper read at the Ohio Valley Sociological Society, South Bend, Indiana, 1967.
37. HUNT, R. G.: "Socio-cultural Factors in Mental Disorder." *Behavioral Science* 14:96-106, 1959.
38. HUSEN, T.: "La Validite des Interviews par Rapport a l'Age, au Sexe et a la Formation des Interviewers." *Travail Humain* 17:60-67, 1954.
39. HUTCHINSON, B.: "The Social Grading of Occupations in Brazil." *British Journal of Sociology* 8:176-189, 1957.
40. LANGNER, T. S.: "Psychophysiological Symptoms and the Status of Women in Two Mexican Communities," in J. M. Murphy and A. H. Leighton (eds.): *Approaches to Cross-Cultural Psychiatry.* New York: Cornell University Press, 1965, pp. 360-392.
41. LESSER, G. S., AND KANDEL, D.: Cross-Cultural Research: Advantages and Problems. Harvard University: Laboratory of Human Development. Unpublished paper.
42. LINDZEY, G.: *Projective Techniques and Cross-Cultural Research.* New York: Appleton-Century-Crofts, pp. 191-192.
43. LINZ, J., AND DE MIGUEL, A.: "Within-nation Differences and Comparisons: The Eight Spains," in R. L. Merritt and S. Rokkan (eds.): *Comparing Nations.* New Haven: Yale University Press, 1966, pp. 267-319.
44. LITTLE, A.: "An Expectancy Estimate of Hospitalization Rates for Mental Illness in England and Wales." *The British Journal of Sociology* 16:221-231.

101

45. MALZBERG, B.: "Mental Disease Among the Native and Foreign-born White Population of New York State, 1939-1941." *Mental Hygiene* 39:545-563.

46. MALZBERG, B. AND LEE, E: Migration and Mental Disease. New York: Social Science Research Council, 1956.

47. MARTIN, F. M.: "Some Subjective Aspects of Social Stratification," in D. V. Glass (ed.): *Social Mobility in Britain*. London: Routledge and Kegan Paul, Ltd., 1954, pp. 51-75.

48. MEZEY, A. G.: "Psychiatric Aspects of Human Migrations." *International Journal of Social Psychiatry* 5:245-260, 1960.

49. MEZEY, A. G.: "Personal Background, Emigration and Mental Disorder in Hungarian Refugees." *Journal of Mental Science* 106:618-627, 1960.

50. MICHEL, A.: "Comparative Data Concerning the Interaction in French and American Families." *Journal of Marriage and the Family* 29:337-344.

51. MITCHELL, R. E.: "Survey Materials Collected in the Developing Countries: Sampling, Measurement, and Interviewing Obstacles to Intra- and International Comparisons." *International Social Science Journal* 17:665-685, 1965.

52. MOSER, C. A., AND HALL, J. R.: "The Social Grading of Occupations," in D. V. Glass (ed.): *Social Mobility in Britain*. London: Routledge and Kegan Paul, Ltd., 1954, pp. 22-50.

53. MURPHY, H. B. M., WITTKOWER, E. D., FRIED, J., AND ELLENBERGER, H.: "A Cross-cultural Survey of Schizophrenic Symptomatology." The *International Journal of Social Psychiatry* 9:237-249, 1963.

54. MURPHY, J. M., AND HUGHES, C. C.: "The Use of Psychophysiological Symptoms as Indicators of Disorder among Eskimos," in J. M. Murphy and A. H. Leighton (eds.): *Approaches to Cross-Cultural Psychiatry*. New York: Cornell University Press, 1965, pp. 108-160.

55. MYERS, J. K., BEAN, L. L., AND PEPPER, M. P.: "Social Class and Psychiatric Disorders: A Ten-year Follow-up." *Journal of Health and Human Behavior* 6:74-79, 1965.

56. ODEGAARD, O.: "Emigration and Insanity." *Acta Psychologica et Neurologica,* Suppl. 4, 1932.

57. OHMURA, M., AND SAWA, H.: "Taylor's Anxiety Scale in Japan." *Psychologia* 1:123-126, 1957.

58. OSGOOD, C. E.: "On the Strategy of Cross-National Research into Subjective Culture." *Social Science Information* 6:5-37, 1967.

59. PETERSEN, W.: Survey Ambiguities. Berkeley: University of California, Department of Sociology. Unpublished paper.

60. PRINCE, R., AND MOMBOUR, W.: "A Technique for Improving Linguistic Equivalence in Cross-cultural Surveys." The *International Journal of Social Psychiatry* 13:229-237, 1967.

61. PRZEWORSKI, A., AND TEUNE, H.: "Equivalence in Cross-Cultural Research." *Public Opinion Quarterly* 30:551-568, 1966-67.

62. RIIHINEN, O.: The Regional Differentiation of an Industrializing Society. Kuopio, Finland: Unpublished, 1965.

63. ROGLER, L. H., AND HOLLINGSHEAD, A. B.: "Class and Disordered Speech in the Mentally Ill." *Journal of Health and Human Behavior* 2:178-185, 1961.

64. SAFILIOS-ROTHSCHILD, C.: "Socio-cultural Aspects of Psychiatric Practice in Greece." Manuscript, a short summary of which was published in *Transcultural Psychiatric Research* 4:177-178, 1967.

65. SAFILIOS-ROTHSCHILD, C.: "Social Class and Success Stereotypes in Greek and American Cultures." *Social Forces* 45:374-383, 1967.

66. SAFILIOS-ROTHSCHILD, C.: "A Comparison of Power Structure and Marital Satisfaction in Urban Greek and French Families." *Journal of Marriage and the Family* 29:345-352, 1967.

67. SAFILIOS-ROTHSCHILD, C.: "Deviance and Mental Illness in the Greek Family." *Family Process* 7:100-117, 1968.

68. SAFILIOS-ROTHSCHILD, C.: Methodological Problems of Research in an Underdeveloped Country. Unpublished manuscript, 1968.

69. SAFILIOS-ROTHSCHILD, C.: "Sociopsychological Factors Affecting Fertility in Urban Greece: A Preliminary Report." *Journal of Marriage and the Family* 31:599-606, 1969.

70. SAFILIOS-ROTHSCHILD, C.: "A Cross-Cultural Comparison of Sex Roles in Fifteen Societies." *Acta Scandinavica, 1971.*

71. SAVAGE, C., LEIGHTON, A. H., AND LEIGHTON, D. C.: "The Problem of Cross-cultural Iden-
     tification of Psychiatric Disorders," in J. M. Murphy and A. H. Leighton (eds.): *Approaches
     to Cross-Cultural Psychiatry*. New York: Cornell University Press, 1965, p.p. 60-62.
72. SAWYER, J.: "Dimensions of Nations: Size, Wealth and Politics." *American Journal of So-
     ciology* 73:145-172, 1967.
73. SCHEUCH, E. K.: The Use of Survey Research in Cross-Cultural Comparisons. Indian Statis-
     tical Institute, International Social Science Council. Unpublished paper.
74. SCHWARTZ, C. G.: "Perspectives on Deviance—Wives' Definitions of Their Husbands'
     Mental Illness." *Psychiatry* 20:275-291, 1957.
75. SHEATSLEY, P. B.: "An Analysis of Interviewer Characteristics and Their Relationship to
     Performance." *International Journal of Opinion and Attitude Research* 4:473-498, 1950.
76. SMITH, H. L., AND HYMAN, H.: "The Biasing Effect of Interviewer Expectations on Survey
     Results." *Public Opinion Quarterly* 14:491-506, 1950.
77. STYCOS, J. M.: "Further Observations on the Recruitment and Training of Interviewers in
     Other Cultures." *Public Opinion Quarterly* 19:68-78, 1955.
78. STYCOS, J. M.: "Education and Fertility in Puerto Rico." World Population Conference 1965,
     vol. 4. New York: United Nations, 1966.
79. SVALASTOGA, K.: *Social Differentiation*. New York: David McKay Co., Inc., 1965.
80. TSUNG-YI-LIN.: "A Study of the Incidence of Mental Disorder in Chinese and Other Cul-
     tures." *Psychiatry* 16:313-336, 1953.
81. USEEM, J., AND GRIMSHAW, A. D.: "Comparative Sociology." *Social Science Research Council
     Items* 20:46-51, 1966.
82. WARNER, O., AND CAMPBELL, D. T.: "Translating, Working Through Interpreters and the
     Problem of Decentering," in R. Naroll and R. Cohen (eds.): *A Handbook of Method in
     Cultural Anthropology*. New York: American Museum of Natural History, 1969.
83. WHYTE, W. F., AND WILLIAMS, L. K.: Supervisory Leadership: An International Comparison.
     New York State School of Industrial and Labor Relations, Cornell University. Unpublished
     manuscript.
84. WILLIAMS, A. J., JR.: "Interviewer-Respondent Interaction: A Study of Bias in the Information
     Interview." *Sociometry* 27:338-352, 1964.
85. WITTKOWER, E. D., AND FRIED, J.: "Some Problems of Transcultural Psychiatry." *The
     International Journal of Social Psychiatry* 3:245-252, 1958.
86. YARROW, M. R., SCHWARTZ, C. G., MURPHY, H. S., AND DEASY, L. C.: "The Psychological
     Meaning of Mental Illness in the Family." *Journal of Social Issues* 11:12-24, 1955.

Part III

RESEARCH IN
PSYCHIATRIC SOCIOLOGY

INTRODUCTION

Changes in patterns of research over a period of time can provide valuable insights into the nature of a subject-matter specialty. Such is the case with psychiatric sociology. Reconstructing the history of the specialty can focus upon publications, a method that only indirectly reflects interaction among a set of scholars sharing the same interests. A chronological series of publications focused on the same general questions is not, however, necessarily a valid indicator of the existence of a new discipline or specialty. Nonetheless, we have little else on which to base a historical perspective.

Studies of the effects of social factors in the development of mental disorder have appeared since early in this century; a distinctive field of psychiatric sociology did not emerge until much later. Looking instead at organized efforts based on intellectual interaction, it appears more appropriate to place the specialty's beginnings in the United States in the 1930's, with the work of Faris and Dunham[2] comprising the publication which generated significant interaction among sociologists sharing an interest in mental disorder. Since the early 1940's and particularly since 1955, work of this type expanded rapidly.

A considerable bulk of sociological work that has dealt with mental disorder has focused upon the question of social etiology. Broader concerns with psychiatry as a profession and as a social institution, with the organization of mental health care and with patterns of undiagnosed maladjustment of various types, are topics of much more recent origin.

The proportion of effort directly concerned with the etiology of behavior disorders has been eclipsed during the past decade. Despite a long history of social etiological research and considerable investments in such efforts, sociologists have been largely unsuccessful in advancing etiological claims which have sound substantiation. Decreases in available funding, perhaps due to the absence of significant break-throughs, curbed efforts in etiological research. It also appears that many sociologists have become frustrated with the limited conceptual and explanatory "pay-offs" produced by etiological research, coupled with the frustrations of methodological inadequacies. Robins' discussion in Chapter 4 outlines the types of strategies necessary for etiological approximations, but in so doing she indicates the technical complexity of such research, to say nothing of the costs and staffing problems entailed. Thus, we might view social etiological research as requiring an input which is often not equivalent to the outcome, particularly in terms of contributions to broader sociological questions.

The amount of attention paid to etiology among psychiatric sociologists has also been affected by the growing prominence of the labeling perspective discussed in Chapter 3 and the type of research stimulated by that perspective. Among the labeling theorists, Lemert[6] is perhaps most prominent in indicating that research on the initial causes of disordered behavior should be of a much lower priority for sociologists than studies focused on the impact of social reac-

106

tions to the deviant individual whose normality is at issue. Lemert and other labeling theorists seem to be saying that the application of sociological efforts to etiological research promises much less than efforts directed at the study of social reactions. The hoped-for "pay-off" of labeling research is an elucidation of social-psychological processes; by contrast, a focus on discrete aspects of social structure pervades etiological studies. In a sense, therefore, labeling research may be more attractive because its results are more exciting; furthermore, its methodology is far less rigorous. Concomitant with the development of labeling theory, there has been an increasing repudiation of the medical model of behavior disorders. Largely as a result of the influence of Szasz and to a lesser extent, Laing, many sociologists have come to doubt the isolated reality of neuroses and psychoses as "diseases." Instead, these behaviors are being viewed as the products of learning through complex interaction processes, followed by changes in role definition which are implicit in psychiatric labeling and concomitant social rejection. Studies which have indicated that social class differences between the psychiatrist and his patient may determine diagnosis have further contributed to the rejection of the medical model. If abnormal behaviors are viewed primarily as products of definitional events (for example, "mental illness is behavior labeled as such by psychiatrists"), the question of etiology is reoriented to the processing of persons through psychiatric systems. Thus, many labelists generally reject the notion that their efforts should involve etiological research of the traditional type; these pursuits are left for biologists and psychologists.

Developments within the field of psychiatry itself have affected enthusiasm for etiological studies. The diffusion of studies of family processes in relation to various types of mental disorder, such as Laing's research, has led in some quarters to a view of disorders such as schizophrenia as being characteristic of interaction systems rather than characteristic of personality (for example Mishler and Waxler) and has involved the use of sociopsychological research designs of considerable complexity. This etiological research is of a much different nature than the field research designs which characterize etiological studies which have typically been conducted by sociologists. Furthermore, the field of sociology has been overshadowed by other disciplines in this type of family process research. Sophisticated methodologies and theories with a strong social-interactional thrust have been developed within the subgroup of psychiatrists who are primarily concerned with family therapy, as documented in the quarterly journal, *Family Process*.

Furthermore, etiological research requires access to patients. This frequently calls for the maintenance of interdisciplinary relations between psychiatrists and sociologists. A not-so-subtle quality of intellectual imperialism characterizes some quarters of psychiatric research. This orientation globally defines psychiatry as "the science of human behavior" which sometimes involves "laying claim" to sociological theories and methods. This in turn is conducive to the attitude in etiological research of "who needs the sociologist?" Such an attitude is reinforced by the results of the aforementioned psychiatric research on family processes,/which has considerable potential input into sociological models of the family. Furthermore, while most earlier cooperative efforts seem to reflect the sociologists' acceptance of psychiatry's legitimacy, much of the literature on labeling questions this legitimacy and sees psychiatry as a dangerous agency of social control. This may have closed some of the doors necessary for the involvement of sociologists in etiological research.

It is, however, incorrect to posit insurmountable barriers between the disciplines of sociology and psychiatry. Instead, it appears that psychiatry currently views sociology as a potentially valuable resource for research focused on questions *other than those concerned with etiology.* The community mental health movement has challenged the field of psychiatry with an elaborate mandate that calls not only for a broadening of treatment activities but also an attack on pathogenic features of community life. As is evidenced in our companion volume, *Sociological Perspectives on Community Mental Health,* there are numerous roles available to the sociologist within the community mental health movement. However, almost none of these positions involves etiological research which, for unknown reasons, no longer appears necessary to many community psychiatrists. These opportunities for sociological involvement often call for skills within the field that are methodological rather than theoretical, involving such practical activities as setting up data collection systems and conducting evaluation research. Such efforts are beginning to make theoretical contributions, particularly when activities such as evaluation are viewed within the framework of organizational behavior. In any event, it appears that many psychiatrists are much more comfortable with such efforts than they are with sociological studies of etiology or studies of the social processes in psychiatric practice.

Many sociologists have been attracted by the availability of brief instruments for the measurement of psychiatric impairment in general populations where individuals have received neither psychiatric labels nor treatment. Recognizing that the biases most often implicit in psychiatric diagnoses yield population samples that may not represent "true prevalence," a considerable number of studies have appeared which have employed the Langner[4] 22-item index as well as the Leighton[5] 20-item index Health Opinion Survey. Such studies have been focused primarily on the antecedents and correlates of different levels of psychiatric impairment.

While this approach is convenient and the instruments are predictive of a psychiatric diagnosis of impairment, psychiatry's traditional disease categories cannot be employed. What then, is being studied? The methodology lends itself to a comparison of social groups rather than the study of individuals, generating potentially valuable data on psychiatric impairment levels in different social systems and situations. While the 22-item and the Health Opinion Survey indexes offer exciting possibilities for exploring the reasons why persons who are disclosed to be suffering from psychiatric impairment have not been so labeled, this possibility remains to be explored.

For these reasons, the study of causation in contemporary psychiatric sociology is considerably different than it was a decade ago. We do not necessarily lament these changes in emphasis or research strategy. Indeed, much of the contemporary work is characterized by a distinctive sociological flavor that was, in many instances, lacking in previous studies. In a large part, the tradition of research stimulated by the Faris and Dunham effort has been necessarily characterized by a greater concern with sampling and the location of appropriate "cases" than with the testing of significant sociological and sociopsychological theories. Oftentimes such studies show elegance in research design and data collection, but the results are interpreted in an *ad hoc* fashion. This does not justify abandonment of this research interest, however, an integration of the labeling approach with more traditional orientations is definitely needed.

The four chapters presented in this part are a sample of perspectives on four fairly distinctive sets of problems involved in considering etiology. In Chapter 6, Melvin Kohn has launched a frontal attack on the issue of social class and schizophrenia that has played a prominent role in psychiatric sociology for many decades. Much of the recent work on this relationship has been focused upon data which appear to support a process of social selection whereby inadequate social performance, prior to the development of schizophrenia, leads to a preponderance of schizophrenics in the lowest social class.[1,9] This contrasts with the notion that forces in lower class life lead to schizophrenic behavior.[8] Kohn attempts to redirect attention to the latter hypothesis and explore linkages between the components of social class and schizophrenia. He deliberately focuses attention upon the possible relevance of genetic factors in the construction of theory based on social class. This approach is in considerable contrast to the heredity *or* environment dichotomy that has pervaded most sociological literature on this topic. While recognizing that studies which have supported a social selection hypothesis have been carefully designed and conducted, Kohn indicates that data from studies of social class and family life create a pressing argument which cannot be ignored. Kohn's implication is that psychiatric sociologists have seemed more interested in dismissing the etiological relevance of social class. Longitudinal studies of social class and schizophrenia which provide adequate tests of these etiological hypotheses are yet to be fully reported. It will indeed be regrettable if the new generation of psychiatric sociologists fail to heed the argument presented by Kohn and assume that we have achieved an adequate understanding of the relationship that exists between social class and schizophrenia.

The sociological nature of depression and its social etiology is the topic of Chapter 7 by Pauline Bart. There is a growing body of evidence to indicate that depression may be the most prevalent of the psychiatric disorders. The attention it has received from sociologists, however, has been minimal. Bart speculates on this omission, indicating that perspectives which view mental disorders as products of social disintegration are probably inadequate to deal with depression. Her research experience leads to the hypothesis that depression may be related to "over-integration" rather than disintegration. After reviewing a number of

109

explanations for depression, Bart hypothesizes that depression is a possible consequence of role loss, presenting data from her own study of depression among middle-aged women. The observations provided by Bart demonstrate what can be learned when the researcher makes a concerted effort to become acquainted with the phenomena under study. It is evident from Bart's conclusions that depression deserves much greater attention by sociologists, particularly in terms of isolating the characteristics of social structure that may contribute to its prevalence as a "symptom choice."

In Chapter 8, Henslin and Campbell focus upon behaviors that may sometimes accompany or terminate depression: attempted and completed suicides. These authors undertake to examine methodological problems affecting research on suicide and to offer some potential solutions. Their own research experiences lead them to reject the use of official statistics in research on the causes of suicide. Instead, they urge the study of the sociology of suicide statistics, for instance, research focused on decision-making processes of coroners and other public officials which lead to different types of suicide rates. They further focus upon the inadequacy of previous attempts to explain suicide, pointing out the range of different variables that have been introduced in this quest. They then introduce suggestions for focusing upon the role of "meanings" in the study of suicide.

In addition to elucidating the sociology of suicide, this chapter has broader implications for methodology in psychiatric sociology. The nature of the dependent variable, that is, defining operationally what we will seek to explain, is a frequent problem. Suicide provides an interesting example of a behavior disorder which is handled both by legal and medical authorities. The unreliability of suicide statistics in determining "true prevalence" demonstrates that definitional processes are usually acts of social behavior rather than scientific decisions. These authors clearly demonstrate, however, that it may be a mistake to cast aside official definitions as being irrelevant on the basis that they are invalid. Instead, the study of such rates and their construction has considerable potential for broadening our understanding of processes of social control.

Throughout this book several references are made to the use of measures of undiagnosed psychiatric impairment. In Chapter 9, Reinhardt and Gray present the findings of a study which employs the Langner 22-item index specifically designed to explore the relationship between anomia and psychiatric impairment. Reinhardt and Gray carefully analyze the concept of anomia as an index of social integration, concluding that social participation may be an empirical referent for at least a portion of the concept. This study relates to several points made previously in this book. First, the study of Reinhardt and Gray meets Weinberg's plea in Chapter 2 for continued exploration of the hypothesis that social isolation may have an etiological bearing on mental illness. Second, their effort reflects attempts to deal with the problems of research strategy discussed by Robins in Chapter 4. Due to its cross-sectional nature, this study cannot isolate the temporal sequence of anomia and psychiatric impairment; it is reasonable to argue that either could precede the other. Through skilled manipulation of the data, however, the authors are able to cast some new light on the Durkheimian question concerning the relationship that exists between social integration and individual behavior.

Perhaps of more pertinence is Reinhardt and Gray's explicit attempt to deal with factors that may intervene between social class and psychiatric impairment, the "mechanisms" of social class influence emphasized by Kohn in Chapter 6. Their findings complement the earlier results reported by Langner and Michael[4] that the same degree of stress leads to greater impairment in the lower class than is true in the other social classes. Reinhardt and Gray's data indicate that anomia may have a greater impact in the upper classes than in the lower classes. They offer the provocative speculation that this may be due to the "abnormality of anomia in the upper classes as contrasted to its commonality in the lower classes." This study sets the stage for the reanalysis of data from numerous studies which include measures of both psychiatric impairment and social integration.

This set of chapters is not intended to cover the topic in terms of etiological studies conducted and reported by psychiatric sociologists. Each of the chapters does, however, highlight a distinctive problem affecting etiological research and each points to research topics which deserve further exploration. As in Part I, once again we find support for the proposition that there need not be a disjuncture between earlier efforts in psychiatric sociology and emerging themes in theory and research.

REFERENCES

1. DUNHAM, H. W.: *Community and Schizophrenia.* Detroit: Wayne State University Press, 1965.
2. FARIS, R. E. L., AND DUNHAM, H. W.: *Mental Disorders in Urban Areas.* Chicago: University of Chicago Press, 1939.
3. LANGNER, T. S.: "The twenty-two item index of psychiatric impairment." *Journal of Health and Human Behavior.* 4:269-274, 1962.
4. LANGNER, T. S., AND MICHAEL, S. T.: *Life Stress and Mental Health.* New York: The Free Press, 1963.
5. LEIGHTON, D. C.: *The Character of Danger.* New York: Basic Books, 1963.
6. LEMERT, E. M.: *Social Pathology.* New York: McGraw Hill, 1951.
7. MISHLER, E., AND WAXLER, N.: *Interaction in Families.* New York: John Wiley, 1968.
8. ROMAN, P. M., AND TRICE, H. M.: *Schizophrenia and the Poor.* Ithaca, New York: Cornell University Press, 1967.
9. TURNER, R. J., AND WAGENFELD, M. O.: "Occupational Mobility and Schizophrenia." *American Sociological Review* 32:104-113, 1967.

CHAPTER 6

Social Class and Schizophrenia: A Critical Review and a Reformulation

MELVIN L. KOHN

My intent in this chapter is to review a rather large and all-too-inexact body of research on the relationship of social class to schizophrenia and to explore its etiological implications. Instead of reviewing the studies one by one, I shall direct myself to general issues and bring in whatever studies are most relevant.* The *raison d'etre* of this review is to organize the evidence around certain central issues and to make use of all studies relevant to those issues. There are no definitive studies in this field, but most of them contribute something to our knowledge when placed in perspective of all the others. For an alternative approach, deliberately limited to those few studies that meet the reviewers' standards of adequacy, Mishler and Scotch[79] would be useful. Dunham[23] has recently argued for a more radical alternative; he disputes the legitimacy of using epidemiological data to make the types of social psychological inference I attempt here and insists that epidemiological studies are relevant only to the study of how social systems function.†

It hardly need be stressed that my way of selecting these issues and my evaluation of the studies represent only one person's view of the field and would not necessarily be agreed to by others.

Before I get to the main issues, I should like to make four prefatory comments:

(1) When I speak of schizophrenia, I shall generally be using that term in the broad sense in which it is usually employed in the United States, rather than in the more limited sense used in much of Europe. The classic definition of

---

*This chapter is an amalgam of two previously published papers [57,59] that the editors and I thought might usefully be brought together into one entity.

†Some other useful reviews and discussions of issues in this field are: Dunham;[19,21] Felix and Bowers;[30] Clausen,[10,12] Hollingshead;[47] Sanua;[107] Roman and Trice;[97] and the Dohrenwends.[18]

schizophrenia[4] considers it to be a group of disorders whose "fundamental symptoms consist of disturbances of association and affectivity, the predilection for fantasy as against reality, and the inclination to divorce oneself from reality." In common with most American investigators, I use the term to refer to those severe functional disorders marked by disturbances in reality relationships and concept formation.[98] I follow American rather than European usage, not because I think it superior, but because it is the usage that has been employed in much of the relevant research. Any comparative discussion must necessarily employ the more inclusive, even if the cruder, term.

(2) I shall generally not be able to distinguish among various types of schizophrenia, for the data rarely enable one to do so. This is most unfortunate; one should certainly want to consider "process" and "reactive" types of disturbance separately,[35] to distinguish between paranoid and nonparanoid, and to take account of several other possibly critical distinctions.

Worse yet, I shall at times have to rely on data about an even broader and vaguer category than schizophrenia—severe mental illness in general, excluding only the demonstrably organic syndromes. I shall, however, do this sparingly and emphasize studies that focus on schizophrenia.

(3) Social classes will be defined as aggregates of individuals who occupy broadly similar positions in the hierarchy of power, privilege, and prestige.[128] In dealing with the research literature, I shall treat occupational position, or occupational position as weighted somewhat by education, as a serviceable index of social class for urban society. I shall not make any distinction, since the data hardly permit my doing so, between the concepts "social class" and "socioeconomic status." And I shall not hesitate to rely on less than fully adequate indices of class when relevant investigations have employed them.

(4) Much of what I shall do in this essay will be to raise doubts and come to highly tentative conclusions from inadequate evidence. This is worth doing because we know so little and the problem is so pressing. Genetics does not seem to provide a complete explanation, and, I take it from Kety's critical reviews,[53, 54] biochemical and physiological hypotheses have thus far failed to stand the test of replication. Of all the social variables that have been studied, those related to social class have yielded the most provocative results.* Thus, inadequate as the following data are, they must be taken seriously.

It must be emphasized, however, that there are exceedingly difficult problems in interpreting the data that I am about to review. The indices are suspect, the direction of causality is debatable, the possibility that one or another alternative interpretation makes more sense than the one I should like to draw is very real indeed. These problems will all be taken up shortly; first, though, I should like to lay out the positive evidence for a meaningful relationship between class and schizophrenia.

---

*For appraisals of the evidence about other social variables and about intersocietal differences in rates of schizophrenia, cf. Eaton and Weil;[25] Mishler and Scotch;[79] Demerath;[16] Goldhamer and Marshall;[39] Lin;[74] and Leighton and Lambo.[70]

114

EVIDENCE ON THE POSSIBLE RELATIONSHIP
OF SOCIAL CLASS TO RATES OF SCHIZOPHRENIA

Most of the important epidemiological studies of schizophrenia can be viewed as attempts to resolve problems of interpretation posed by the pioneer studies, Faris and Dunham's[29] ecological study of rates of schizophrenia for the various areas of Chicago and Clark's[8,9] study of rates of schizophrenia at various occupational levels in that same city. Their findings were essentially as follows:

Faris and Dunham: The highest rates of first hospital admission for schizophrenia are in the central city areas of lowest socioeconomic status, with diminishing rates as one moves toward higher-status peripheral areas. The pattern is most marked for paranoid schizophrenia, least so for catatonic, which tends to concentrate in the foreign-born slum communities. Unfortunately, subsequent studies in smaller cities dealt with too few cases to examine the distribution of separable types of schizophrenia as carefully as did Faris and Dunham.

Clark: The highest rates of schizophrenia are found in the lowest status occupations, with diminishing rates as one goes to higher status occupations.

The concentration of high rates of mental disorder, particularly of schizophrenia, in the central city *areas* of lowest socioeconomic status has been confirmed in a number of American cities—Providence, Rhode Island[29] Peoria, Illinois; Kansas City, Missouri;[109] St. Louis, Missouri;[15,90,109] Milwaukee, Wisconsin;[109] Omaha, Nebraska; Worcester, Massachusetts;[36] Rochester, New York;[34] and Baltimore, Maryland.[55] The two ecological studies done in European cities—Sundby and Nyhus's[121] study of Oslo, Norway and Hare's[44] of Bristol, England—are in substantial agreement too. There are some especially difficult problems in interpreting the ecological findings present in these studies which I shall not discuss here because most of the later and crucial evidence comes from other modes of research. The problems inherent in interpreting ecological studies are discussed in Robinson,[94] and in Clausen and Kohn.[13]

The concentration of high rates of mental disorder, particularly of schizophrenia, in the lowest status *occupations* has been confirmed again and again. The studies conducted by Hollingshead and Redlich[49] in New Haven, Connecticut, and by Srole and his associates[118] in midtown, New York City, are well-known examples; a multitude of other investigations in the United States have come to the same conclusion.[23,32,33,71,76,105,124] Relevant, too, are some early studies whose full significance was not appreciated until later.[42,84,85] One puzzling partial-exception comes from Jaco's[51] study of Texas. He finds the highest incidence of schizophrenia among the unemployed, but otherwise a strange, perhaps curvilinear relationship of occupational status to incidence. It may be that so many of his patients were classified as unemployed, rather than according to their pre-illness occupational status, that the overall picture is distorted. Moreover, Svalastoga's reanalysis of Strömgren's data for northern Denmark is consistent, as are the Leightons'[68] data for "Stirling County," Nova Scotia, Ode-

115

gaard's[85, 87] for Norway, Stein's[119] for two sections of London, Brooke's for England and Wales, Lin's[75] for Taiwan, and Stenbäck and Achte's[120] for Helsinki.

But there are some exceptions. Clausen and I[14] happened across the first, when we discovered that for Hagerstown, Maryland, there was no discernible relationship between either occupation or the social status of the area and rates of schizophrenia. In that paper, the data on occupational rates were incompletely reported. Although we divided the population into four occupational classes, based on United States Census categories, we presented the actual rates for only the highest and lowest classes, leading some readers to conclude, erroneously, that we had divided the population into only two occupational classes. In fact, the average annual rates of first hospital admission for schizophrenia, per 100,000 population aged 15 to 64 were:

(a) professional, technical, managerial, officials and proprietors: 21.3
(b) clerical and sales personnel: 23.8
(c) craftsmen, foremen, and kindred workers: 10.7
(d) operatives, service workers, and laborers: 21.7

Our measures of occupational mobility, to be discussed later, were based on movement among the same four categories. On a re-examination of past studies, we discovered a curious thing: the larger the city, the stronger the correlation between rates of schizophrenia and these indices of social class. In the metropolis of Chicago, the correlation is large, and the relationship is linear: the lower the social status, the higher the rates. In cities of 100,000 to 500,000 (or perhaps more), the degree of correlation is smaller and not so linear: it is more a matter of a concentration of cases in the lowest socioeconomic strata, with not so much variation among higher strata. When you get down to a city as small as Hagerstown—36,000—the degree of correlation disappears.

Subsequent studies in a number of different places have confirmed our generalization. Sundby and Nyhus,[121] for example, showed that Oslo, Norway, manifests the typical pattern for cities of its 500,000 size: a high concentration in the lowest social stratum, little variation above. Hollingshead and Redlich's[49] data on new admissions for schizophrenia from New Haven, Connecticut, show that pattern, too. There is substantial evidence, too, for our conclusion that socioeconomic differentials disappear in areas of small population.[7, 43]

I think one must conclude that the relationship of socioeconomic status to schizophrenia has been demonstrated only for urban populations. Even for urban populations, a linear relationship of socioeconomic status to rates of schizophrenia has been demonstrated only for the largest metropolises. The evidence, though, that there is an unusually high rate of schizophrenia in the lowest socioeconomic strata of urban communities seems to me to be nothing less than overwhelming. The proper interpretation of why this is so, however, is not so unequivocal.

116

THE DIRECTION OF CAUSALITY

One major issue in interpreting the Faris and Dunham, the Clark, and all subsequent investigations concerns the direction of causality. Rates of schizophrenia in the lowest socioeconomic strata could be disproportionately high either because conditions of life in those strata are somehow conducive to the development of the illness or because people from higher social strata who become schizophrenic suffer a decline in status. Or, of course, it could be some of both. Discussions of this issue have conventionally gone under the rubric of the "drift hypothesis," although far more is involved.

The drift hypothesis was first raised as an attempt to explain away the Faris and Dunham findings. The argument was that in the course of their developing illness, those suffering from schizophrenic illnesses tend to drift into lower status areas of the city. It is not that more cases of schizophrenia are produced in these areas, but that such individuals are products of another area and then end up at the bottom of the heap by the time they are hospitalized; thus, they are counted as having come from the bottom of the heap.

When the Clark study appeared, the hypothesis was easily enlarged to include drift from higher to lower-status occupations. In its broadest formulation, the drift hypothesis asserts that high rates of schizophrenia in the lowest social strata come about because people from higher classes who become schizophrenic suffer a decline in social position as a consequence of their illness. In some versions of the hypothesis, it is further suggested that those with schizophrenic illness from smaller locales tend to migrate to the lowest status areas and occupations of large metropolises; this would result in an exaggeration of rates there and a corresponding underestimation of rates for the place and class from which they come.

One approach to this problem has been to study the histories of social mobility of individuals who exhibit symptoms characteristic of schizophrenia. Unfortunately, the evidence is inconsistent. Three studies indicate that schizophrenics have been downwardly mobile in occupational status. Evidence that schizophrenics have been downwardly mobile in *occupational* status has been presented by Schwartz;[112] *Lystad;*[77] and Turner.[123] In addition, there has been some debatable evidence that the ecological concentration of schizophrenia has resulted from the migration of unattached men into the high-rate areas of the city. Three other studies indicated, however that individuals with schizophrenia were not downwardly mobile in occupational status. Evidence to this effect is presented by Hollingshead and Redlich;[48] Clausen and Kohn;[14] and Dunham.[22] Evidence that the ecological concentration of schizophrenia has not resulted from in-migration or downward drift is presented by LaPouse and associates;[66] Hollingshead and Redlich;[48] and, if I interpret his data correctly, by Dunham.[23] Some of these studies do not compare the experiences of the individuals with schizophrenia to those of normal persons from comparable social backgrounds.

Those that do are nevertheless inconclusive—either because the comparison group was not well chosen, or because the city in which the study was done was too small to have a concentration of schizophrenia in the lowest social class. Since no study is definitive, any assessment must be based on a subjective weighing of the strengths and weaknesses of them all. My assessment is that the weight of this evidence clearly indicates either that schizophrenic individuals have been no more downwardly mobile (in fact, no less upwardly mobile) than other people from the same social backgrounds, or at minimum, that the degree of downward mobility is insufficient to explain the high concentration of schizophrenia in the lowest socioeconomic strata.

There is another and more direct way of looking at the question, however, but from this perspective the question is still unresolved. The reformulated question focuses on the social class origins of particular individuals with this psychosis; it asks whether the occupations of their fathers are concentrated in the lowest social strata. If they are, that is clear evidence in favor of the hypothesis that lower class status is conducive to schizophrenia. If they are not, class still might matter for schizophrenia—it might, for example, be a matter of stress experienced by lower-class adults, rather than of the experience of being born and raised in the lower class. Certainly the explanation that would require the fewest assumptions would be the drift hypothesis.

The first major study to evaluate the evidence from this perspective argued in favor of lower-class origins being conducive to mental disorder, although not necessarily to schizophrenia in particular. Srole and his associates[118] found, in their study of midtown New York, that rates of mental disorder do correlate with parents' socioeconomic status, even if not as strongly as with the subjects' own socioeconomic status. But then Goldberg and Morrison[38] found that although the occupations of male schizophrenic patients admitted to hospitals in England and Wales show the usual concentration of cases in the lowest social class, their fathers' occupations do not. Since this study was addressed specifically to schizophrenia, the new evidence seemed more directly in point. One might quarrel with some aspects of the study—the index of social class is debatable, for example, and data are lacking for 25 per cent of the originally drawn sample— but this is much too good a study to be taken lightly. Nor can one conclude that the situation in England and Wales is different from that in the United States, for Dunham[23, 24] and Rinehart[92] report that two segments of Detroit show a pattern similar to that reported by Goldberg and Morrison.

There is yet one more study to be considered, however, and this the most important one of all, for it offers the most complete data about class origins, mobility, and the eventual class position of schizophrenic men. Turner and Wagenfeld,[124] in a study of Monroe County (Rochester), New York, discovered a remarkable pattern: rates of first treatment for schizophrenia are disproportionately high, both for patients of lowest occupational status and for patients whose fathers had lowest occupational status, but these are by and large not the same patients. Some of those whose fathers were in the lowest occupational category had themselves moved up and some of those ending in the lowest occupational category had come from higher class origins. Thus, there is evidence both for the proposition that lower-class origins are conducive to schizophrenia and for the proposition that most lower-class schizophrenics come from higher socioeconomic origins. Downward social mobility does not explain the class-schizophrenia relationship, but it does contribute to that relationship.

How much downward mobility is there, and how does it occur? Turner and Wagenfeld's data indicate that the absolute amount of downward mobility is almost negligible: 36 per cent of the schizophrenic individuals in their sample have fallen and 35 per cent have risen from their fathers' occupational levels, for a net decline of less than one-tenth of a step on a seven-point occupational scale. In the general population, although, there has been a net rise of nearly one-half step on the same seven-point scale. Thus, one could say that, *relative to the general population,* those diagnosed as being schizophrenic have been downwardly mobile. More precisely, they have lagged behind the general population in not rising above their fathers' occupational levels. This has happened, not because they lost positions they had once achieved, but because many of them failed ever to achieve as high an occupational level as do most men of their social class origins.

These findings argue strongly against a simple drift hypothesis. It is not, as some have argued, that we have erroneously rated men at lower than their usual socioeconomic levels because we have classified them according to their occupations at time of hospitalization, after they have suffered a decline in occupational position. It is likely, though, that a more sophisticated drift hypothesis applies—that some people genetically, constitutionally or otherwise predisposed to schizophrenia show debilitating effects at least as early as the time of their first jobs, because they are never able to achieve the occupational levels that might be expected of them. If so, the possibilities of some interaction between genetic predisposition and early social circumstances are very real indeed. It is also possible that downward social mobility has occurred in earlier generations—that because of genetic or other defects, the parents and grandparents have also failed to achieve as high a position as might have been expected of them. I defer consideration of this possibility until I have discussed the evidence for a genetic component in schizophrenia.

For the present, I think it can be tentatively concluded that despite what Goldberg and Morrison found for England and Wales, the weight of evidence lies against the drift hypotheses providing a sufficient explanation of the class-schizophrenia relationship. In all probability, lower-class families produce a disproportionate number of schizophrenic off-spring, although perhaps by not so large a margin as one would conclude from studies that rely on their occupational attainments.

The Adequacy of Indices

The adequacy of indices is another major issue in interpreting the Faris and Dunham, the Clark, and all subsequent investigations. Most of these studies are based on hospital admission rates, which may not give a valid picture of the true incidence of schizophrenia. Studies that do not rely on hospital rates encounter other and perhaps even more serious difficulties, with which we shall presently deal.

The difficulty with using admission rates as the basis for computing rates of schizophrenia is that lower-class psychotics may be more likely to be hospitalized, and if hospitalized to be diagnosed as schizophrenic, especially in public hospitals. Faris and Dunham tried to solve this problem by including patients admitted to private as well as to public mental hospitals. This was insufficient because, as later studies have shown,[52] some people who suffer serious mental disorder never enter a mental hospital.

Subsequent studies have attempted to do better by including more and more social agencies in their search for cases; Hollingshead and Redlich[49] in New Haven, and Jaco[51] in Texas, for example, have extended their coverage to include everyone who enters any sort of treatment facility—Jaco going so far as to question all the physicians in Texas. This is better, but clearly the same objections hold in principle. Furthermore, Srole and his associates[118] have demonstrated that there are considerable social differences between people who have been treated, somewhere, for mental illness, and severely impaired people, a large proportion of them schizophrenic, who have never been to any sort of treatment facility. So we must conclude that using treatment of any sort as an index of mental disorder is suspect.

The alternative is to go out into the community and examine everyone, or a representative sample of everyone, yourself. This has been done by a number of investigators, for example Essen-Möller[27, 28] in Sweden, Srole[118] in New York, the Leightons[68] in Nova Scotia. They have solved one problem, but have run into three others.

The first is that most of these investigators have found it impossible to classify schizophrenia reliably, and have had to resort to larger and vaguer categories—severe mental illness, functional psychosis, and so forth. For some purposes, this may be justified. For our immediate purposes, it is exceedingly unfortunate.

Second, even if one settles for such a concept as mental illness, it is difficult to establish criteria that can be applied reliably and validly in community studies.[17] For all its inadequacies, hospitalization is at least an unambiguous index, and one can be fairly certain that people who are hospitalized are disturbed. But how does one interpret the Leightons'[69] estimate that about a third of their population suffer significant psychiatric impairment, or Srole's[118] that almost a quarter of his are impaired?

The third problem in community studies is that it is so difficult to secure data on the incidence of mental disturbance that most studies settle for prevalence data.[62] That is, instead of ascertaining the number of new cases arising in various population groups during some period of time, they count the number of people currently ill at the time of the study. This latter measure—prevalence—is inadequate because it reflects not only incidence but also duration of illness. As Hollingshead and Redlich[49] have shown, duration of illness, insofar as it incapacitates, is highly correlated with social class. Clearly, what is needed is repeated studies of the population, to pick up new cases as they arise and thus to establish true incidence figures. The crucial problem, of course, is to develop reliable measures of mental disorder, for without that our repeated surveys will measure nothing but the errors of our instruments. In the meantime, we have to recognize that prevalence studies use an inappropriate measure that exaggerates the relationship of socioeconomic status to mental disorder.

So, taken all together, the results of the studies of class and schizophrenia are hardly definitive. They may even all wash out—one more example of inadequate methods leading to premature, false conclusions. I cannot prove otherwise. Yet I think the most reasonable interpretation of all these findings is that they point to something real. Granted that there is not a single definitive study in the lot, the weaknesses of one are compensated for by the strengths of some other, and the total edifice is probably much stronger than one would conclude from knowing only how frail its component parts are. A large number of complementary studies all seem to point to the same conclusion: that rates of mental disorder, particularly of schizophrenia, are highest at the lowest socioeconomic levels, at least in moderately large cities, and this probably is not just a matter of drift, inadequate indices, or some other artifact of the methods we use. In all probability, more schizophrenia is actually produced at the lowest socioeconomic levels. At any rate, let us take that as a working hypothesis and explore the question further. Assuming that more incidence of schizophrenia occurs at lower socioeconomic levels, let us examine why.

ALTERNATIVE INTERPRETATIONS* OF THE CLASS-SCHIZOPHRENIA RELATIONSHIP

Many discussions of the class-schizophrenia relationship have focused on interpretations that, in effect, explain away its theoretical significance. This is obviously true of those interpretations that consider the relationship to be artifactual, the result of methodological error. It is equally true of interpretations, of which the drift hypothesis is prototypic, that assert that schizophrenic patients are found disproportionately in lower social classes because of the impairment they have suffered or because of some characterological defect of nonsocial origin. The social statuses of schizophrenics may tell us something about how they fare in society but little or nothing about what produces the psychosis.

---

*Although some of the interpretations discussed in this section have been addressed to mental illness in general, they are equally applicable to schizophrenia.

Others argue that class matters for schizophrenia, not because lower-class conditions of life are conducive to the development of the disorder, but because a person's social class position affects other people's perceptions of and reactions to his behavior. One such interpretation asserts that psychiatric and other authorities are especially prone to stigmatize and hospitalize lower-class people: they victimize the powerless. This interpretation is a logical outgrowth of Goffman's[37] analysis of the "moral career of the mental patient," which sees hospitalization as the end-product of a "funnel of betrayal," with the psychiatrist as a major culprit. Goffman deals only in passing with the possibility of class differences in the likelihood of victimization, but some of his followers argue that psychiatrists are especially prone to hospitalize lower-class people and to diagnose them as schizophrenic; middle-class people are spared, if not hospitalization, at least the stigma of the diagnosis. Similar, though more subtle, explanations focus on the processes by which families, employers, police, and others come to label some deviant behaviors as mentally disordered, thereby setting in motion complex changes in social expectation and self-conception that sometimes eventuate in hospitalization.

Scheff[108] presents a cogent formulation of the labeling theory approach as applied to mental disorder. But Gove[41] marshals evidence that this approach is based on assumptions that are inconsistent with what is known: principally, that people strongly resist seeing deviant behavior as being mentally disordered; the pressures, instead, are to interpret even grotesque behavior as somehow normal and situationally explainable. From this point of view, the class-schizophrenia relationship documents the discriminatory readiness of many people to see signs of mental disorder in lower-class behavior.

Even interpretations that accord a primary causal significance to social structural conditions have generally de-emphasized the importance of social class, *per se*. Faris and Dunham, for example, did not take class very seriously in interpreting their data. From among the host of variables characteristic of the high-rate areas of Chicago, they focused on such things as high rates of population turnover and ethnic mixtures and hypothesized that the really critical thing about the high-rate areas was the degree of social isolation they engendered. Two subsequent studies, one by Jaco[50] in Texas, the other by Hare[44] in Bristol, England, are consistent in that they, too, show a correlation between rates of schizophrenia and various ecological indices of social isolation. The only study that directly examines the role of social isolation in the lives of schizophrenics, however, seems to demonstrate that while social isolation may be symptomatic of developing illness, it does not play an important role in etiology.[60]

Several other possibilities have been suggested, some supported by intriguing, if inconclusive, evidence. One is that it is not socioeconomic status as such that is principally at issue, but rather social integration; the Leightons[68] have produced plausible evidence for this interpretation. Another is that the high rates of schizophrenia found in lower-class populations are a consequence of especially high rates for lower-class members of some "ethnic" groups who happen to be living in areas where other ethnic groups predominate. In their study in Boston, for example, Schwartz and Mintz[111] showed that Italian-Americans living in predominantly non-Italian neighborhoods have very high rates of schizophrenia, while those living in predominantly Italian neighborhoods do not; the former group contributes disproportionately to the rates for lower-class neighborhoods. Wechsler and Pugh[126] extended this interpretive model to suggest that rates should be higher for any persons living in a community where persons of their social attributes are in a minority. Their analysis of Massachusetts towns provides some surprisingly supportive data.

Other interpretations focus on the occupational component of socioeconomic status. Odegaard[85] showed that rates of schizophrenia are higher for some occupations that are losing members and lower for some that are expanding; in recent times, declining occupations have generally been of lower status. Alternatively, some investigators see the key in discrepancies that exist between schizophrenic individuals occupational aspirations and achievements, arguing that the pivotal fact is not that they have achieved so little but that they had wanted so much more.[56,83,88]

These several interpretations are, for the most part, consistent with existing data and must be acknowledged to be plausible. But they largely neglect the most straightforward possibility of all—that social class is related to schizophrenia primarily because the conditions of life built into lower social class position are conducive to that disorder.

I think it is time to devote a larger portion of our efforts to devising and testing formulations about how and why lower-class conditions of life might contribute to schizophrenia. The remainder of this essay is devoted to presenting one such formulation. It is necessarily tentative, for it is based on seriously incomplete information; at critical places, there is no directly pertinent evidence and I can only speculate.

THE INFLUENCE OF GENETICS AND STRESS ON SCHIZOPHRENIA

To try to explain the relationship of class to schizophrenia without bringing other variables into play would be extremely difficult. One would be hard pressed to resolve the apparent contradiction that, although lower-class conditions of life appear to be conducive to causing schizophrenia, the vast majority of lower-class people never develop the disorder.[97] When, however, one brings genetics and stress into consideration, the task becomes more manageable. It is no longer necessary to find in class itself an explanation of schizophrenia. Instead, the interpretive task is to explain how social class fits into an equation that includes genetics, probably stress, and undoubtedly other, as yet unrecognized, factors.

Genetics

Recent studies of monozygotic twins and of adopted children demonstrate that although genetics alone cannot provide a sufficient explanation of schizophrenia, some genetic mechanism is almost undoubtedly involved.* Geneticists do not agree on what is inherited—whether it be a vulnerability specifically to schizophrenia, a vulnerability to mental disorder more generally, or even a type of personality structure. Nor is it certain whether the mode of genetic transmission is monogenic or polygenic. Important as these questions may be, they can for our immediate purposes be passed over; all that need be accepted is that genetics plays some substantial role in schizophrenia.

One could argue, in fact, that genetics explains why *class* is related to schizophrenia. If there is a heritable component in schizophrenia, there must have been higher than usual rates of the disorder among the parents and grandparents of those with the psychosis. Moreover, since schizophrenia is debilitating, there would have been downward social mobility in earlier generations. Thus, those with schizophrenia could come disproportionately from lower-class families, not because the conditions of life experienced by lower-class people have pernicious effects, but because there is a concentration of genetically susceptible people in the lower social classes.

These processes of "multigenerational drift" may well contribute to the increased probability of schizophrenia for people of lower class position. The question, though, is whether there could have been *enough* downward mobility attributable to the genetically induced disabilities of earlier generations to account for the heightened incidence of schizophrenia found today in the lower social classes.

Since there are no data about the mobility rates of parents and grandparents of schizophrenics, one can only come to a tentative appraisal based on data about the individuals themselves. As indicated earlier, schizophrenic men have not actually declined from their fathers' occupational levels, but they have lagged behind the general population in not rising above those levels. These data make it doubtful that there could have been enough of an increase in genetic susceptibility to schizophrenia in the lower social classes, even over several generations, to account for all, or even the major part of the class-schizophrenia relationship. It would take a large amount of downward mobility, not just a moderate lag in upward mobility, to have a pronounced effect on the total amount of genetic susceptibility in the lower social classes. Moreover, data based on the occupational histories of schizophrenic patients probably exaggerate the amount of occupational lag that occurred in earlier generations; it can reasonably be assumed that the parents and grandparents were, on the average, less disturbed and therefore less likely to lag in mobility than were the schizophrenic patients themselves. Fi-

---

*For a comprehensive assessment of the genetic evidence, see Rosenthal.[103] Other valuable discussions are to be found in Rosenthal;[100] [102] Kringlen;[63] [64] Slater;[116] and Shields.[114] For discussions of the mode of genetic transmission, cf. Gottesman and Shields;[40] Rosenthal;[103] and Heston.[46]

nally, we need not assume that all deficits in occupational attainment are genetically induced or have genetic consequences. In all probability, genetically induced, intergenerational social mobility has contributed to, but falls far short of explaining, the higher incidence of schizophrenia in the lower social classes.

Stress

Investigators of the role of stress in schizophrenia face a perplexing problem in defining and indexing stress.[18, 67, 113] A narrow conception would have that term apply only to externally induced events that can be assumed to be psychically painful to virtually everyone who experiences them. Such a conception achieves rigor at the price of excluding from its purview those traumas that may have been self-induced, as well as all those traumas that are painful for some people but not for everyone. It also excludes such real, if self-defined, misfortunes as failure to attain a longed-for goal. In fact, the only experiences that can be assumed to be externally induced and to be painful for everyone are such crises as serious illness, death of close relatives, hunger, and loss of one's job; and even these misfortunes may not be equally painful to all who experience them. But broader conceptions of stress are also problematic. At the extreme, if any event that produces subjectively experienced pain in some individual is considered to be stressful, formulations that attribute to stress a causal role in schizophrenia become tautological.

Research workers have for the most part dealt with this dilemma by, explicitly or implicitly, defining as stressful those events that usually are externally induced and that can be expected to be painful to most people who experience them. Such events occur with greater frequency at lower social class levels: people at the bottom of the class hierarchy experience great economic insecurity and far more than their share of serious ill health, degradation, and the afflictions attendant on inadequate, overcrowded housing, often in over-populated, underserviced areas.

Is stress conducive to schizophrenia? A definitive study would require direct, rather than inferential, measurement of stress; a research design that takes social class explicitly into account; and, of course, an adequate index of schizophrenia. Not surprisingly, no study meets all these criteria. Therefore, one can make only a tentative overall appraisal, recognizing that some pertinent studies do not index stress as well as we should like, others do not explicitly control social class, and some are addressed to mental disorder in general rather than specifically to schizophrenia.

My appraisal of the research evidence is based primarily on the studies by Rogler and Hollingshead,[96] Brown and Birley,[6] Birley and Brown,[3] Langner and Michael,[65] and Etinger[26]. These studies do indicate that stress is associated with the occurrence of schizophrenia. Moreover, Rogler and Hollingshead show that the relationship between stress and schizophrenia does not simply reflect the high levels of stress prevalent in the lower social classes. From their investigation of schizophrenics and matched controls in the lowest social class of San Juan,

Puerto Rico, they report that during the year before the onset of symptoms, the individuals experienced notably greater stress than did the control subjects. One note of caution however: the Rogler-Hollingshead study is based on schizophrenic individuals who are married or living in stable consensual unions. On the basis of this stability, one would assume them to be predominantly suffering from "reactive" schizophrenia—precisely the group whom clinical studies describe as having had normal childhood social experiences, good social adjustment, and extreme precipitating circumstances. So these findings may apply only to reactive schizophrenia, not to process schizophrenia. It may also be that some of the stress they experienced resulted from their already disordered behavior. Still, Rogler and Hollingshead present a strong case that externally induced stress is important for some types of schizophrenia. Even when judged by the harsh standards of life of the San Juan slums, the stresses that preceded the onset of schizophrenia were unusually severe.

As with genetics, one must reverse the question and ask whether stress can explain the relationship of class to schizophrenia. The Rogler-Hollingshead study cannot help us here, for it is limited to one social class. Unfortunately for our purposes, the only study that does provide data for all levels of social class, that by Langner and Michael, is addressed to mental disorder in general rather than specifically to schizophrenia. This study is nevertheless germane, for it indicates that at any given level of stress, people of lower social class position are more likely to become mentally disturbed than are people of higher social class position. In fact, the more sources of stress, the greater the class difference in the proportion of people who manifest psychotic symptoms. The implication is that the relationship of class to mental disorder (hence, if we may extrapolate, to schizophrenia) is not attributable to the amount of stress that people endure. There must also be important class differences in how effectively people deal with stress.

Part of the explanation for lower-class people dealing less effectively with stress may be that the stress-producing situations they face are less alterable by individual action than are those encountered by people of higher social class position. Many of the stresses they encounter arise from economic circumstances over which few individuals have much control, lower-class individuals least of all. Moreover, lower-class people have little money or power to employ in coping with the consequences of stress. It also appears[18] that fewer institutional resources are available to them, either for escaping stressful situations or for mitigating the consequences of stress. Finally, there is reason to believe that lower-class conditions of life limit people's *internal* resources for dealing with stress.[18] Pertinent, too, are the discussions by Brewster Smith[117] of "the competent self," by Foote and Cottrell[31] of "interpersonal competence," and by Phillips[89] of "social competence."

While recognizing that all these factors may make it difficult for lower-class people to deal effectively with stress, my formulation emphasizes only one: that their conditions of life may impair lower-class people's internal resources. I shall argue, more generally, that these life conditions may adversely affect people's ability to deal, not only with situations that by my limited definition are stressful, but also with many other dilemmas and uncertainties in a rapidly changing, complex society.

A critic might contend that an adequate explanation of the class-schizophrenia relationship can be formulated without taking internal resources into account—that one can explain the heightened incidence of schizophrenia in the lower social classes as resulting from a combination of greater genetic vulnerability, greater exposure to stress, and lesser external resources for dealing with stress. Present evidence is too scanty for a definitive judgment, but I think this formulation is too narrow; it ignores too much of what we know about the social psychology of class. And so I shall devote much of the remainder of this essay to laying out the reasons for believing that lower-class conditions of life may adversely affect people's internal resources for dealing with stressful, problematic, or complex situations, and for believing that such impairment may be important in the schizophrenic process.

CLASS, FAMILY, AND SCHIZOPHRENIA

If internal resources for dealing with complex and stressful situations are at issue, then that primary socializing institution, the family, is probably somehow involved. The many studies of the role of the family in the development of schizophrenia are pertinent here, even although most of them have been addressed to a question quite different from ours. The purpose of these investigations has generally been to find some pattern of interpersonal relationship unique to the families where schizophrenia is present. To the best of my knowledge, although, no well-controlled study has shown a substantial difference between the patterns of parent-child relationship characteristic of families that produce schizophrenic offspring and those characteristic of ordinary lower-class families.* This sweeping conclusion is based on my inability, and that of others who have reviewed the research literature, to find a single study that finds important differences in patterns of parent-child relationship between schizophrenics and normal persons of lower social class background. Several well-controlled studies find an absence of difference.[61,81,96]

From a traditional, single factor perspective, two interpretations of this negative finding are possible. One would be that the family plays no important part in the genesis of schizophrenia. This interpretation holds that the patterns of parent-child relationship typical of schizophrenia-producing families merely reflect those of the lower social classes from which schizophrenics disproportionately come, without having been instrumental in the disorder.†

---

*For a comprehensive, if now dated, review of research on family and schizophrenia, see Sanua,[107] and also the introduction to, and references included in, Kohn and Clausen;[61] the discussion and references in Mishler and Waxler,[80] and pp. 140-163 of Rosenbaum.[98]

†For an incisive review of research on class and family, see Bronfenbrenner.[5] For references to studies completed since Bronfenbrenner's review, and to studies done outside the United States, see Kohn.[58]

The alternative interpretation would assert that the family does play a critically differentiating role in schizophrenia, but that the statistical evidence is not yet in. From this point of view, most well-controlled studies have been too limited in focus. They have dealt with such relatively concrete aspects of family life as the overall pattern of role-allocation, parental bestowal of warmth and affection, and disciplinary practices, but have missed more subtle interpersonal processes that recent clinical investigations have emphasized. In support of this position are indications that lower-class families with schizophrenic offspring, although no different from other lower-class families in role-patterning, may manifest disturbed, even pathological, patterns of communication.[2, 98] Future studies may show clear and convincing evidence of important differences between schizophrenia-producing families and ordinary families of lower social class position.

There is, however, a third possible interpretation. Instead of looking to the family for a total explanation of schizophrenia, this interpretation attempts only to explain how lower-class families may contribute to the disorder in genetically vulnerable people who are subject to great stress. From this perspective, the family is important for schizophrenia, not because their family experiences have differed in some presently undisclosed manner from those of other people of lower social class background, but precisely because they have been similar. If this be the case, there is no reason to restrict our interest to processes that are unique to the family, such as its particular patterns of role allocation. We should expand our focus to include, even to emphasize, processes that the family shares with other institutions—notably, those processes that affect people's ability to perceive, to assess, and to deal with complexity and stress. One implication is that it is not only the social class of one's parental family, but also one's adult social class position, that matters for schizophrenia. This point is often overlooked, particularly in discussions of the drift hypothesis.

I suggest that the family is important principally because of its strategic role in transmitting to its offspring conceptions of social reality that parents have learned from their own experience. In particular, many lower-class families transmit to their offspring an orientational system too limited and too rigid for dealing effectively with complex, changing, or stressful situations. By orientation (or orientational system), I mean conceptions of the external world and of self that serve to define men's stance toward reality. This point of view is, I believe, consonant with recent psychiatric thinking about the family and schizophrenia, which emphasizes those communicational and cognitive processes in schizophrenia-producing families that contribute to the schizophrenic's difficulties in interpreting social reality. Especially relevant here is the work of Lyman Wynne and his associates.[115,129, 329] Additionally the work of Mishler and Waxler;[80] Bateson and his associates,[1] and Schuham[110] will be helpful.

What is new is the assertion that these conceptions of reality, far from being unique to families whose offspring become schizophrenic, are widely held in the lower social classes, and in fact arise out of the very conditions of life experienced by people in these segments of society.

SOCIAL CLASS AND CONCEPTIONS OF REALITY

My hypothesis is that the constricted conditions of life experienced by people in lower social classes foster conceptions of social reality so limited and so rigid as to impair their ability to deal resourcefully with the problems and the stress. Although speculative, this hypothesis is a direct extrapolation from what is known about the relationship between social class and conceptions of reality.[104] My own research[58] indicates that the lower a man's social class position, the more likely he is to value conformity to external authority and to believe that such conformity is all that his own capacities and the exigencies of the world allow. In particular, the lower one's social class position, the more likely is his orientational system to be marked by a rigidly conservative view of man and his social institutions, fearfulness and distrust, and a fatalistic belief that one is at the mercy of forces and people beyond one's control, often, beyond one's understanding.

One need not argue that this orientational system is held by all lower-class people, or that lower-class people hold these beliefs and values to the exclusion of others, more characteristic of higher social classes[78,95] It does seem to be well established, though, that these conceptions of social reality are most prevalent at the bottom of the social hierarchy.

The existence of class differences in beliefs and values is hardly accidental, nor even cultural in the sense employed by "culture of poverty" theorists who see lower-class orientations as something handed down from generation to generation independently of current social conditions.* The principal issue, as I see it, is not whether there are class differences in values, orientation, and cognitive style, but whether the lower-class orientational systems, once transmitted from parents to children, are amenable to change. My data show that if there is a discrepancy between early family experience and later educational and occupational conditions, the latter are likely to be more influential.[58] The practical implications of this finding are as important as they are obvious: the most efficacious way to alleviate the burdens of lower social classes is not by therapy, resocialization, or other efforts to teach middle-class values and orientation, but rather by changing the social conditions to which people are subject.

It is necessary to consider that the nature of social class embodies such basic dissimilarities in conditions of life that subjective reality depends upon where people are differentially situated in the social hierarchy. Lower-class conditions of life allow little freedom of action and give one little reason to feel in control of his fate. To be a member of the lower class is to be insufficiently educated, to

---

*For a systematic statement of the culture of poverty thesis, see Lewis.[72] For critiques of this and related concepts, see Valentine;[125] Roach and Gursslin;[93] and Rossi and Blum.[104]

work at a job of little substantive complexity, under conditions of close supervision, and with little leeway to vary a routine flow of work. These are precisely the conditions that narrow one's conception of social reality and reduce one's sense of personal efficacy.[58]

There is, then, ample evidence to prove that class differences in conditions of life are capable of producing differences in conceptions of social reality. But do these differences in orientation contribute to class differences in schizophrenia? There are three reasons for thinking that they might.

The first is a consideration of theoretical strategy. Instead of searching aimlessly among the innumerable correlates of social class for one or another that might help explain its relationship to schizophrenia, I think it is strategic to look at what underlies the social psychology of class: members of different social classes, by virtue of enjoying (or suffering) different conditions of life, come to see the world differently—to develop different conceptions of social reality, aspirations, hopes and fears, and different conceptions of what is desirable. Class differences in orientation are an important bridge between social conditions and psychological functioning.

The second reason for thinking that orientations are pertinent is that our analysis of the interrelationship of class, genetics, and stress points to the desirability of taking into account any factor that might have an important bearing on class differences in how effectively people are able to deal with stressful or problematic situations. It seems to me that the orientation towards conformity that is characteristic of the lower social classes is less adequate for dealing with such situations than is the self-directed orientation more prevalent at higher social class levels.

Admittedly, the characteristically lower-class orientational system, molded as it is by actual conditions, may often be useful. It is, for example, attuned to the occupational demands that lower-class people must meet; a self-directed stance would probably bring few rewards and might easily lead to trouble. Moreover, participant-observation studies of lower-class life[73, 127] make it vividly apparent that, in an environment where one may be subject to diverse and often unpredictable risks of exploitation and victimization, this perspective may serve other protective functions as well. It is a way of keeping one's guard up. It provides a defensive strategy for people who are vulnerable to forces they cannot control.

But there are times when a defensive posture invites attack, and there are times when the assumption that one is at the mercy of forces beyond one's control—even where justified—leaves one all the more defenseless. A class orientational system predicated on conforming to the dictates of authority sees social reality too simply and fearfully to permit taking advantage of options that might otherwise be open. It is too inflexible for precisely those problematic and stressful circumstances that most require subtlety, flexibility, and a perceptive understanding of larger social complexities.

130

The third reason is that orientations—conceptions of reality—are fundamental to schizophrenia. Fearful, inflexible reactions to threat are integral to the schizophrenic experience. One reason for the disproportionately high incidence of schizophrenia at lower social class levels may be that schizophrenic disorders build on conceptions of reality firmly grounded on the experiences of these social classes.

CONCLUSION

My proposed formulation attempts to bring genetics, stress, and the conditions of life attendant on social class position into one coherent interpretation of schizophrenia. The thrust of the argument is that the conditions of life experienced by people of lower social class position tend to impair their ability to deal resourcefully with problems and stress. Such impairment would be unfortunate for all who suffer it, but would not in itself result in schizophrenia. In conjunction with a genetic vulnerability to schizophrenia and the experience of great stress, though, such impairment could well be disabling. Since both genetic vulnerability and stress appear to occur disproportionately at lower social class levels, people in these segments of society may be in triple jeopardy.

In trying to make my point forcefully, I may have exaggerated statistical tendencies, making it seem as if class differences in orientational systems were differences in kind rather than in degree. I hope it is clear from the general argument, though, that all the relevant variables—genetics, stress, conceptions of reality—must be seen as probabilistic; the formulation depends on the joint occurrence of these necessary conditions.

How would one test such a formulation? Since the formulation posits that schizophrenia is produced by the interaction of genetic vulnerability, stress, and the disabilities attendant on a conformist orientation, a rigorous test clearly requires that all three elements be considered together. I speak of interaction in its precise statistical sense: the relevance of any of the three factors depends on the strength of the other two. It may also be that the critical threshold for each of the factors depends on the strength of the other two. If, for example, the genetic predisposition is exceptionally strong, less stress may be required;[101] if there is exceedingly great stress, perhaps only minimal genetic vulnerability will be sufficient;[26] if a person's orientation is strongly conformist, even moderately stressful situations may overwhelm him. These possibilities, and the numerous variations they imply, suggest that my model may be only a simple prototype of a family of models. Fortunately, research designed to test any one of them can assess the others as well, for they are all based on the interplay of the same three factors.

If the effects of genetics, stress, and orientation were assumed to be additive, we could test any of them by comparing schizophrenics to nonschizophrenics of the same social class on that factor alone. But with an interactive model of the type I have proposed, a single-factor comparison is inadequate. Since no one

131

factor could produce schizophrenia except in combination with the others, it would be possible for *all* members of a given social class to surpass the threshold for any factor, provided they did not exceed thresholds for the others. Thus, an absence of difference between those with evidence of the disorder and those symptom free of the same class level on any of the factors in the model is no disproof of the pertinence of that factor. Correspondingly, finding a difference provides *prima facie* evidence that the factor is pertinent to schizophrenia, but no proof that its place in the model has been correctly established. An important corollary is that different factors may distinguish schizophrenics from nonschizophrenics in different social classes.

To be concrete: the correlations between class and the pertinent facets of orientation range from 0.13 to 0.38. If one took the moderate size of these correlations to imply that many lower-class people do not hold a conformist orientation, he would predict substantial differences in orientation between those lower-class people who do and those who do not become schizophrenic. But I interpret the moderate correlations between class and orientation to mean that a conformist orientation is widely held at lower social class levels and is far from absent, although less widely held, at higher social class levels. I would therefore predict little or no difference in orientation between those in the lower-class who are schizophrenic and those who are not. From either perspective, we should expect schizophrenics and nonschizophrenics in the lower-class to differ most decidedly in genetic vulnerability, perhaps also in exposure to stress, and least of all in orientation. Since present evidence suggests that the correlation between class and orientation is greater than that between class and genetics, or than that between class and stress, the differences that exist between schizophrenic people and those who show no evidence of the psychosis should center more and more on orientation at increasingly higher social class levels.

REFERENCES

1. BATESON, G., JACKSON, D., HALEY, J. AND WEAKLAND, J.: "Toward a Theory of Schizophrenia." *Behavioral Science* 1:251-264, 1956.
2. BEHRENS, M. I., ROSENTHAL, A. J., AND CHODOFF, P.: "Communication in Lower Class Families of Schizophrenics: II. Observations and Findings." *Archives of General Psychiatry* 18:689-696, 1968.
3. BIRLEY, J. L. T., AND BROWN G. W.: "Crises and Life Changes Preceding the Onset or Relapse of Acute Schizophrenia: Clinical Aspects." *British Journal of Psychiatry* 116:327-333, 1970.
4. BLEULER, E.: *Dementia Praecox or the Group of Schizophrenias.* New York: International Universities Press, 1950.
5. BRONFENBRENNER, U.: "Socialization and Social Class Through Time and Space," in Eleanor E. Maccoby, Theodore M. Newcomb, and Eugene L. Hartley (eds.): *Readings in Social Psychology.* New York: Henry Holt and Company, 1958, pp. 400-425.
6. BROWN, G. W., AND BIRLEY, J. L. T.: "Crises and Life Changes and the Onset of Schizophrenia." *Journal of Health and Social Behavior* 9:203-214, 1968.
7. BUCK, C., WANKLIN J. M., AND HOBBS, G. E.: "An Analysis of Regional Differences in Mental Illness." *The Journal of Nervous and Mental Disease* 122:73-79, 1955.

8. CLARK, R. E.: "The Relationship of Schizophrenia to Occupational Income and Occupational Prestige." *American Sociological Review* 13:325-330, 1948.
9. CLARK, R. E.: "Psychoses, Income, and Occupational Prestige." *American Journal of Sociology* 54:433-440, 1949.
10. CLAUSEN, J. A.: *Sociology and the Field of Mental Health.* New York: Russell Sage Foundation, 1956.
11. CLAUSEN, J. A.: "The Ecology of Mental Illness." Symposium on Social and Preventive Psychiatry. Walter Reed Army Medical Center, Washington, D. C.:97-108, 1957.
12. CLAUSEN, J. A.: "The Sociology of Mental Illness," in Robert K. Merton, Leonard Broom, and Leonard S. Cottrell, Jr. (eds.): *Sociology Today, Problems and Prospects.* New York: Basic Books, 1959, Pp. 485-508.
13. CLAUSEN, J. A., AND KOHN, M. L.: "The Ecological Approach in Social Psychiatry." *American Journal of Sociology* 60:140-151, 1954.
14. CLAUSEN, J. A., AND KOHN, M. L.: "Relation of Schizophrenia to the Social Structure of a Small City," in Benjamin Pasamanick (ed.): *Epidemiology of Mental Disorder.* Washington, D. C.: American Association for the Advancement of Science, 1959, Pp. 69-94.
15. DEE, W. L. J.: "An Ecological Study of Mental Disorders in Metropolitan St. Louis." Unpublished M. A. thesis. Washington University, 1939.
16. DEMERATH, N. J.: "Schizophrenia Among Primitives," in Arnold M. Rose (ed.): *Mental Health and Mental Disorder.* New York: W. W. Norton, 1955, Pp. 215-222.
17. DOHRENWEND, B. P., AND DOHRENWEND, B. S.: "The Problem of Validity in Field Studies of Psychological Disorder." *Journal of Abnormal Psychology* 70:52-69, 1965.
18. DOHRENWEND, B. P., AND DOHRENWEND, B. S.: *Social Status and Psychological Disorder: A Causal Inquiry.* New York: John Wiley and Sons, 1969.
19. DUNHAM, H. W.: "Current Status of Ecological Research in Mental Disorder." *Social Forces* 25:321-326, 1947.
20. DUNHAM, H. W.: "Social Psychiatry." *American Sociological Review* 13:183-197, 1948.
21. DUNHAM, H. W.: "Some Persistent Problems in the Epidemiology of Mental Disorders." *American Journal of Psychiatry* 109:567-575, 1953.
22. DUNHAM, H. W.: "Social Class and Schizophrenia." *American Journal of Orthopsychiatry* 34:634-642, 1964.
23. DUNHAM, H. W.: *Community and Schizophrenia: An Epidemiological Analysis.* Detroit: Wayne State University Press, 1965.
24. DUNHAM, H. W., PHILLIPS P., AND SRINIVASAN, B.: "A Research Note on Diagnosed Mental Illness and Social Class." *American Sociological Review* 31:223-227, 1966.
25. EATON, J. W., AND WEIL, R. J.: *Culture and Mental Disorders: A Comparative Study of the Hutterites and Other Populations.* Glencoe, Illinois: Free Press, 1955.
26. EITINGER, L.: *Concentration Camp Survivors in Norway and Israel.* Oslo: Universitetsforlaget, 1964.
27. ESSEN-MÖLLER, E.: "Individual Traits and Morbidity in a Swedish Rural Population." *Acta Psychiatrica et Neurologica Scandinavica.* Supplement 100:1-160, 1956.
28. ESSEN-MÖLLER, E.: "A Current Field Study in the Mental Disorders in Sweden," in Paul H. Hoch and Joseph Zubin (eds.): *Comparative Epidemiology of the Mental Disorders.* New York: Grune and Stratton, 1961, Pp. 1-12.
29. FARIS, R.E.L., and DUNHAM, H.W.: *Mental Disorders in Urban Areas: An Ecological Study of Schizophrenia and Other Psychoses.* Chicago: University of Chicago Press, 1939.
30. FELIX, R.H., and BOWERS, R.O.: "Mental Hygiene and Socio-Environmental Factors." *The Milbank Memorial Fund Quarterly* 26:125-147, 1948.
31. FOOTE, N., AND COTTRELL, JR., L.S.: *Identity and Interpersonal Competence: A New Direction in Family Research.* Chicago: University of Chicago Press, 1955.
32. FRUMKIN, R.M.: "Occupation and Major Mental Disorders," in Arnold Rose (ed.): *Mental Health and Mental Disorders.* New York: W.W. Norton, 1955, Pp. 136-160.
33. FUSON, W.M.: "Research Note: Occupations of Functional Psychotics." *American Journal of Sociology* 48:612-613, 1943.
34. GARDNER, E.A., AND BABIGIAN, H.M.: "A Longitudinal Comparison of Psychiatric Service to Selected Socioeconomic Areas of Monroe County, New York." *American Journal of Orthopsychiatry* 36: 818-828, 1966.
35. GARMEZY, N.: "Process and Reactive Schizophrenia: Some Conceptions and Issues," in

133

Martin M. Katz, Jonathan O. Cole, and Walter E. Barton (eds.): *The Role and Methodology of Classification in Psychiatry and Psychopathology.* Washington, D.C.: U.S. Government Printing Office (PHS Publication No. 1584), 1965, Pp. 419-466.

36. GERARD, D.L., AND HOUSTON, L.G.: "Family Setting and the Social Ecology of Schizophrenia." *Psychiatric Quarterly* 27:90, 101, 1953.
37. GOFFMAN, E.: "The Moral Career of the Mental Patient." *Psychiatry* 22:123-142, 1959.
38. GOLDBERG, E.M., AND MORRISON, S.L.: "Schizophrenia and Social Class." *British Journal of Psychiatry* 109:785-802, 1963.
39. GOLDHAMER, H., AND MARSHALL, A.W.: *Psychosis and Civilization: Two Studies in the Frequency of Mental Disease.* Glencoe, Illinois: The Free Press, 1953.
40. GOTTESMAN, I.I., AND SHIELDS, J.: "A Polygenic Theory of Schizophrenia." *Proceedings of the National Academy of Sciences* 58:199-205, 1967.
41. GOVE, W.R.: "Societal Reaction as an Explanation of Mental Illness: An Evaluation." *American Sociological Review* 35:873-884, 1970.
42. GREEN, H.W.: Persons Admitted to the Cleveland State Hospital, 1928-37. Cleveland Health Council, 1939.
43. HAGNELL, O.: *A Prospective Study of the Incidence of Mental Disorder.* Stockholm: Syenska Bokförlaget, 1966.
44. HARE, E.H.: "Mental Illness and Social Conditions in Bristol." *Journal of Mental Science* 102:349-357, 1956.
45. HARE, E.H.: "Family Setting and the Urban Distribution of Schizophrenia." *Journal of Mental Science* 102:753-760, 1956.
46. HESTON, L.L.: "The Genetics of Schizophrenic and Schizoid Disease." *Science* 167:249-256, 1970.
47. HOLLINGSHEAD, A.B.: "Some Issues in the Epidemiology of Schizophrenia." *American Sociological Review* 26:5-13, 1961.
48. HOLLINGSHEAD, A.B., AND REDLICH, F.C.: "Social Stratification and Schizophrenia." *American Sociological Review* 19:302-306, 1954.
49. HOLLINGSHEAD, A.B., AND REDLICH, F.C.: *Social Class and Mental Illness: A Community Study.* New York: John Wiley and Sons, 1958.
50. JACO, E.G.: "The Social Isolation Hypothesis and Schizophrenia." *American Sociological Review* 19:567-577, 1954.
51. JACO, E.G.: *The Social Epidemiology of Mental Disorders: A Psychiatric Survey of Texas.* New York: Russell Sage Foundation, 1960.
52. KAPLAN, B., REED, R.B., AND RICHARDSON, W.: "A Comparison of the Incidence of Hospitalized and Nonhospitalized Cases of Psychosis in Two Communities." *American Sociological Review* 21:472-479, 1956.
53. KETY, S.S.: "Recent Biochemical Theories of Schizophrenia," in Don D. Jackson (ed.): *The Etiology of Schizophrenia.* New York: Basic Books, 1960, Pp. 120-145.
54. KETY, S.S.: "Biochemical Hypotheses and Studies," in Leopold Bellak and Laurence Loeb (eds.): *The Schizophrenic Syndrome.* New York: Grune and Stratton, 1969, Pp. 155-171.
55. KLEE, G.D., SPIRO, E., BAHN, A.K., AND GORWITZ, K.: "An Ecological Analysis of Diagnosed Mental Illness in Baltimore," in Russell R. Monroe, Gerald D. Klee, and Eugene B. Brody (eds.): *Psychiatric Epidemiology and Mental Health Planning.* Psychiatric Research Report No. 22. Washington: The American Psychiatric Association, 1967, Pp. 107-148.
56. KLEINER, R.J. AND PARKER, S.: "Goal-Striving, Social Status, and Mental Disorder: A Research Review." *American Sociological Review* 28:189-203, 1963.
57. KOHN, M.L.: "Social Class and Schizophrenia: A Critical Review," in David Rosenthal and Seymour S. Kety (eds.): *The Transmission of Schizophrenia.* Oxford: Pergamon Press, 1968, Pp. 155-173.
58. KOHN, M.L.: *Class and Conformity: A Study in Values.* Homewood, Illinois: The Dorsey Press, 1969.
59. KOHN, M.L.: Class, Family, and Schizophrenia: A Reformulation." *Social Forces,* 1972.
60. KOHN, M.L., AND CLAUSEN, J.A.: "Social Isolation and Schizophrenia." *American Sociological Review* 20:265-273, 1955.
61. KOHN, M.L., AND CLAUSEN, J.A.: "Parental Authority Behavior and Schizophrenia." *American Journal of Orthopsychiatry* 26:297-313, 1956.

62. KRAMER, M.: "A Discussion of the Concepts of Incidence and Prevalence as Related to Epidemiologic Studies of Mental Disorders." *American Journal of Public Health* 47:826-840, 1957.

63. KRINGLEN, E.: "Schizophrenia in Twins: An Epidemiological-Clinical Study." *Psychiatry* 29:172-184, 1966.

64. KRINGLEN, E.: *Heredity and Environment in the Functional Psychoses: An Epidemiological-Clinical Twin Study.* Oslo: Universitetsforlaget, 1967.

65. LANGNER, T.S., AND MICHAEL, S.T.: *Life Stress and Mental Health.* New York: The Free Press of Glencoe, 1963.

66. LAPOUSE, R., MONK, M.A., AND TERRIS, M.: "The Drift Hypothesis and Socioeconomic Differentials in Schizophrenia." *American Journal of Public Health* 46:978-986, 1956.

67. LAZARUS, R.S.: *Psychological Stress and the Coping Process.* New York: McGraw-Hill, 1966.

68. LEIGHTON, D.C., HARDING, J.S., MACKLIN, D.B., MACMILLAN, A.M., AND LEIGHTON, A.H.: *The Character of Danger: Psychiatric Symptoms in Selected Communities.* New York. Basic Books, 1963.

69. LEIGHTON, D.C., HARDING, J.S., HUGHES, C.C., AND LEIGHTON, A.H.: "Psychiatric Findings of the Stirling County Study." *American Journal of Psychiatry* 119:1021-1026, 1963.

70. LEIGHTON, A.H., LAMBO, T.A., HUGHES, C.C., LEIGHTON, D.C., MURPHY, J.M., AND MACKLIN, D.B.: *Psychiatric Disorder among the Yoruba.* Ithaca: Cornell University Press, 1963.

71. LEMKAU, P., TIETZE, C., AND COOPER, M.: "Mental-Hygiene Problems in an Urban District: Second Paper." *Mental Hygiene* 26:100-119, 1942.

72. LEWIS, O.: *LaVida: A Puerto Rican Family in the Culture of Poverty—San Juan and New York.* New York: Random House, 1965.

73. LIEBOW, E.: *Tally's Corner: A Study of Negro Streetcorner Men.* Boston: Little, Brown and Company, 1960.

74. LIN, T. "A Study of the Incidence of Mental Disorder in Chinese and other Cultures." *Psychiatry* 16:313-336, 1953.

75. LIN, T., RIN, H., YEH, E.K., HSU, C.C., AND CHU, H.M.: "Mental Disorders in Taiwan, Fifteen Years Later: A Preliminary Report," in William Caudill and Tsung-yi Lin (eds.): *Mental Health Research in Asia and the Pacific.* Honolulu: East-West Center Press, 1969, Pp. 66-91.

76. LOCKE, B.Z., KRAMER, M., TIMBERLAKE, C.E., PASAMANICK, B., AND SMELTZER, D.: "Problems of Interpretation of Patterns of First Admissions to Ohio State Public Mental Hospitals for Patients with Schizophrenic Reactions," in Benjamin Pasamanick and Peter H. Knapp (eds.): *Social Aspects of Psychiatry.* The American Psychiatric Association (Psychiatric Research Reports No. 10), 1958, Pp. 172-196.

77. LYSTAD, M.H.: "Social Mobility Among Selected Groups of Schizophrenic Patients." *American Sociological Review* 22:288-292, 1957.

78. MILLER, S.M.: "The American Lower Classes: A Typological Approach," in Frank Riessman, Jerome Cohen, and Arthur Pearl (eds.): *Mental Health of the Poor.* New York: The Free Press of Glencoe, 1964, Pp. 139-154.

79. MISHLER, E.G., AND SCOTCH, N.A.: "Sociocultural Factors in the Epidemiology of Schizophrenia: A Review." *Psychiatry* 26:315-351, 1963.

80. MISHLER, E.G., AND WAXLER, N.E.: "Family Interaction Processes and Schizophrenia: A Review of Current Theories." *Merrill-Palmer Quarterly of Behavior and Development* 11:269-315, 1965.

81. MISHLER, E.G., AND WAXLER, N.E.: *Interaction in Families: An Experimental Study of Family Processes and Schizophrenia.* New York: John Wiley and Sons, 1968.

82. MORRIS, J.N.: "Health and Social Class." *The Lancet* 303-305, 1959.

83. MYERS, J.K., AND ROBERTS, B.H.: *Family and Class Dynamics in Mental Illness.* New York: John Wiley and Sons, 1959.

84. NOLAN, W.J.: "Occupation and Dementia Praecox." (New York) *State Hospitals Quarterly* 3:127-154, 1917.

85. ODEGAARD, O.: "The Incidence of Psychoses in Various Occupations." *International Journal of Social Psychiatry* 2:85-104, 1956.

135

86. ODEGAARD, O.: "Occupational Incidence of Mental Disease in Single Women." *Living Conditions and Health* 1:169-180, 1957.
87. ODEGAARD, O.: "Psychiatric Epidemiology." *Proceedings of the Royal Society of Medicine* 55:831-837, 1962.
88. PARKER, S., AND KLEINER, R.J.: *Mental Illness in the Urban Negro Community*. New York: Free Press, 1966.
89. PHILLIPS, L.: *Human Adaptation and Its Failures*. New York: Academic Press, 1968.
90. QUEEN, S.A.: "The Ecological Study of Mental Disorders." *American Sociological Review* 5:201-209, 1940.
91. RAINWATER, L.: "The Problem of Lower-Class Culture and Poverty-War Strategy," in Daniel P. Moynihan (ed.): *On Understanding Poverty: Perspectives from the Social Sciences*. New York: Basic Books, 1968.
92. RINEHART, J.W.: "On Diagnosed Mental Illness and Social Class." *American Sociological Review* 31:545-546, 1966.
93. ROACH, J.L., AND GURSSLIN, O.R.: "An Evaluation of the Concept 'Culture of Poverty.'" *Social Forces* 45:383-392, 1967.
94. ROBINSON, W.S.: "Ecological Correlations and the Behavior of Individuals." *American Sociological Review* 15:351-357, 1950.
95. RODMAN, H.: "The Lower-Class Value Stretch." *Social Forces* 42:205-215, 1963.
96. ROGLER, L.H., AND HOLLINGSHEAD, A.B.: *Trapped: Families and Schizophrenia*. New York: John Wiley and Sons, 1965.
97. ROMAN, P.M., AND TRICE, H.M.: *Schizophrenia and the Poor*. Ithaca: Cornell University Press, 1967.
98. ROSENBAUM, C.P.: *The Meaning of Madness: Symptomatology, Sociology, Biology and Therapy of the Schizophrenias*. New York: Science House, 1970.
99. ROSENTHAL, A.J., BEHRENS, M.I., AND CHODOFF, P.: "Communication in Lower Class Families of Schizophrenics: I. Methodological Problems." *Archives of General Psychiatry* 18:464-470, 1968.
100. ROSENTHAL, D.: "Problems of sampling and diagnosis in the major twin studies of schizophrenia." *Journal of Psychiatric Research* 1:116-134, 1962.
101. ROSENTHAL, D.: *The Genain Quadruplets: A Case Study and Theoretical Analysis of Heredity and Environment in Schizophrenia*. New York: Basic Books, 1963.
102. ROSENTHAL, D.: "The heredity-environment issue in schizophrenia," in David Rosenthal and Seymour S. Kety (eds.): *The Transmission of Schizophrenia*. Oxford: Pergamon Press, 1968, Pp. 413-427.
103. ROSENTHAL, D.: *Genetic Theory and Abnormal Behavior*. New York: McGraw-Hill, 1970.
104. ROSSI, P.H., AND BLUM, Z.D.: "Class, status, and poverty," in Daniel P. Moynihan (ed.): *On Understanding Poverty: Perspectives from the Social Sciences*. New York: Basic Books, 1968.
105. RUSHING, W.A.: "Two Patterns in the Relationship Between Social Class and Mental Hospitalization." *American Sociological Review* 34:533-541, 1969.
106. SANUA, V.D.: "Sociocultural Factors in Families of Schizophrenics: A Review of the Literature." *Psychiatry* 24:246-265, 1961.
107. SANUA, V.D.: "The Etiology and Epidemiology of Mental Illness and Problems of Methodology: With Special Emphasis on Schizophrenia." *Mental Hygiene* 47:607-621, 1963.
108. SCHEFF, T.J.: *Being Mentally Ill: A Sociological Theory*. Chicago: Aldine, 1966.
109. SCHROEDER, C.W.: "Mental Disorders in Cities." *American Journal of Sociology* 48:40-48, 1942.
110. SCHUHAM, A.I.: "The Double-Bind Hypothesis a Decade Later." *Psychological Bulletin* 68:409-416, 1967.
111. SCHWARTZ, D.T., AND MINTZ, N.L.: "Ecology and Psychosis Among Italians in 27 Boston Communities." *Social Problems* 10:371-374, 1963.
112. SCHWARTZ, M.S.: "The Economic and Spatial Mobility of Paranoid Schizophrenics and Manic Depressives." Unpublished M.A. thesis, University of Chicago, 1946.
113. SCOTT, R., AND HOWARD, A.: "Models of Stress." in Sol Levine and Norman A. Scotch (eds.): *Social Stress*. Chicago: Aldine, 1970, Pp. 259-278.

114. Shields, J.: "Summary of the Genetic Evidence." in David Rosenthal and Seymour S. Kety (eds.): *The Transmission of Schizophrenia*. Oxford: Pergamon Press, 1968, Pp. 95-126.

115. Singer, M.T., and Wynne, L.C.: "Thought Disorder and Family Relations of Schizophrenics: Methodology Using Projective Techniques; Results and Implications." *Archives of General Psychiatry* 12:187-212, 1965.

116. Slater, E.: "A Review of Earlier Evidence on Genetic Factors in Schizophrenia." in David Rosenthal and Seymour S. Kety (eds.): *The Transmission of Schizophrenia*. Oxford: Pergamon Press, 1968, Pp. 15-26.

117. Smith, M.B.: "Competence and Socialization," in John A. Clausen (ed.): *Socialization and Society*. Boston: Little, Brown and Company, 1968, Pp. 270-320.

118. Srole, L., Langner, T.S., Michael, S.T., Opler, M.K., and Rennie, T.A.C.: *Mental Health in the Metropolis: The Midtown Manhattan Study*. New York: McGraw-Hill, 1962.

119. Stein, L.: " 'Social Class' Gradient in Schizophrenia." *British Journal of Preventive and Social Medicine* 11:181-195, 1957.

120. Stenbäck, A., and Achte, K.A.: "Hospital First Admissions and Social Class." *Acta Psychiatrica Scandinavica* 42:113-124, 1966.

121. Sundby, P., and Nyhus, P.: "Major and Minor Psychiatric Disorders in Males in Oslo: An Epidemiological Study." *Acta Psychiatrica Scandinavica* 39: 519-547, 1963.

122. Svalastoga, K.: *Social Differentiation*. New York: David McKay, 1965.

123. Turner, R.J.: "Societal Mobility and Schizophrenia." *Journal of Health and Social Behavior* 9:194-203, 1968.

124. Turner, R.J., and Wagenfeld, M.O.: "Occupational Mobility and Schizophrenia: An Assessment of the Social Causation and Social Selection Hypotheses." *American Sociological Review* 32:104-113, 1967.

125. Valentine, C.A.: *Culture and Poverty: Critique and Counter-Proposals*. Chicago: University of Chicago Press, 1968.

126. Wechsler, H., and Pugh, T.F.: "Fit of Individual and Community Characteristics and Rates of Psychiatric Hospitalization." *American Journal of Sociology* 73:331-338, 1967.

127. Whyte, W.F.: *Street Corner Society: The Social Structure of an Italian Slum*. Chicago: University of Chicago Press, 1943.

128. Williams, R.M., Jr.: *American Society: A Sociological Interpretation*. New York: Knopf, 1951.

129. Wynne, L.C.: "Family Transactions and Schizophrenia: Conceptual Considerations for a Research Strategy," in John Romano (ed.): *The Origins of Schizophrenia*. Amsterdam: Excerpta Medica International Congress Series No. 151, 1967, Pp. 165-178.

130. Wynne, L.C., and Singer, M.T.: "Thought Disorder and Family Relations of Schizophrenics: A Classification of Forms of Thinking." *Archives of General Psychiatry* 9:191-206, 1963.

CHAPTER 7

The Sociology of Depression

PAULINE B. BART

Sociologists, with rare exceptions, have not written about depressive disorders. Schizophrenia, however, has long been an attractive field for investigation, with patterns of admission to hospitals conveniently following the concentric circles first shown by sociologists at the University of Chicago.[35] Admission rates are high in the center of the city, the disorganized areas, and low in the suburbs. Controversies regarding the validity of these statistics still exist. Alcoholism likewise has received a good deal of attention from the sociological discipline. Suicide, which is related to depressive disorders, has been a traditional concern of sociologists, but rarely has it been studied as "the mortality of depressive mental illness."[41] Depression, the disorder or symptom that is most commonly encountered by psychiatrists, has been overlooked. For example, of the four collections of readings in psychiatric sociology which have appeared in the past seven years, only one includes an article on depression. Even in this collection a researcher might not be able to locate information on the topic, since depression is not included in the index, and the article used, Rose's "A Social Psychological Theory of Neurosis," does not mention depression in the title.

In this chapter I first give some reasons for this omission; next, I attempt to integrate psychiatric and sociological theories of depression; and third, I discuss a sociological study of depression.

THE NEGLECT OF DEPRESSION

The first reason for the lack of attention to depression may lie in the "un-American" quality of that mood state. While the theme of Black blues music is unhappiness, the underlying assumption is that people generally feel unhappy, and that this can be a natural state. Some of the music points out the transitory character of this feeling. "You may wake up in the morning with the blues all round your head, but, though you have trouble in mind, and are blue, you won't be blue always/Sun's gonna shine on my backyard someday."

In contrast, Americans are urged to walk "on the sunny side of the street." There is a sense of official optimism. Thus, when people are unhappy, they suffer not only from the affect of sadness itself, but from *experiencing guilt about the feeling.* Whatever the cause of the original depression, *they are unhappy because they are depressed,* and thus suffer from what I term "metadepressions." Since depression is not believed to be a natural state, there must be something the matter with an individual who is unhappy. For example, before Betty Frieden's *Feminine Mystique*[21] was written, some depressed, bored, and trapped housewives who felt guilty about their feelings in the 1950's discovered that it was not a private problem reflecting psychopathology but rather a public issue, that is, a structurally induced motivation common to a large segment of women, that "the American Dream" was, in fact, the American Nightmare. But usually when Americans complain, they are urged to think of their advantages and "blessings." They are often told the homily about the man who felt bad because he had no shoes until he met a man with no feet. In short, the *legitimacy* of the feeling of depression is denied.

Second, sociology has been more concerned with problems stemming from a *lack* of integration into society. The Tocquevillian vision, reflected in the works of Tonnies, Weber, and Simmel, triumphed over the Marxian.[47] The data now available on depression, including the results of the study I report on later in this chapter, suggest that depression is the sickness in the soul of the over-integrated, the conventional, and the believers in tradition.[6,12] It is the illness of those who believed that virtue was rewarded and evil punished, who unlike schizophrenics, trusted and became involved with people, and whose trust was violated.

Who is depressed? Women, traditionally the more conventional of the sexes— the carriers of culture—have a higher rate of depression than men.[41] Middle-aged, middle class, married, never divorced housewives; those women who assumed the traditional roles of wife and mother, have a higher rate of depression than working women or women who have been divorced.

A third reason for the sociological neglect of depression is the data on social class. This evidence is contradictory but it is clear that depression is not particularly characteristic of the poor. Whether it is disproportionately present among the middle and upper class is open to some question, but these strata are certainly not underrepresented.[41] Cohen[12] notes that while schizophrenia is more frequently found among men, members of lower socioeconomic strata, and marginal populations, "among those persons whose group memberships are weakest and most atomistic," depression is frequent among those who "most cohesively identify with their families, kin groups, communities or other significant groupings." "Therefore," he continues, "we find more depression among women, higher socioeconomic strata, traditionalized and tightly knit societal groups, professional people, and suburbanites." In terms of specific social groups, the Hutterites[16] have been found to be depressed.

The strong social cohesion and clear cut expectations which tend to protect Hutterites from having to face the uncertainties of life unaided and without normative guidance, can also be a source of psychological stress. Strong guilt feelings were found in Hutterites who feared that they might be unable to live up to the expectations of their group. Severe depressive moods were the most common psychopathological symptoms in neurotic and psychotic members of the sect [p. 102].

These depressed individuals were generally well integrated into the community; a large per cent of them were leaders, as were their wives. "Hutterites believe that depression is a condition which befalls 'good people.' "

In summary, the distribution of depression can furnish a radical criticism of society. It is entirely congruent with the philosophy of melioristic liberalism that poor people are disproportionately schizophrenic. The solution seems obvious. Remove the very real stresses of poverty and racism, make the poor middle class, culturally and economically, and these mental conditions will be mitigated. But, without denying the very real suffering of those at the bottom of the societal ladder, things are not that simple. For if those segments of society who represent the official norms (or in the case of the Hutterites, a cohesive community) become depressed, those who "believe," who are integrated into or locked into the American scene, then it is possible that the society is not only schizophrenogenic for those left out, but depressenogenic for those let in.

Methodological Problems in Studying Depression

In addition to the more ideological reasons, there are two methodological reasons for the lack of attention paid to depression by sociologists. First, statistics on depression are not as easily available as those on other diagnostic categories. One can find the number of admissions for schizophrenia in psychiatric censuses, but in order to find those for depression, psychotic depression, involutional melancholia, involutional mixed states (depressive and paranoid symptoms), schizoaffective depression, and manic-depression must be found. In addition, patients who have symptoms of depression but have other diagnoses as well should be studied. Even if a researcher wants to gather information on all the various types of depressions, he will find neurotic depression frequently included in a category simply called "neurosis"; some of the other categories are often not listed separately but called "other psychoses." Therefore, most of the studies[17] that have mentioned rates of depression refer only to manic-depressive states.

Furthermore, sociologists studying mental illness have frequently studied admissions to state hospitals, or have studied teaching hospitals affiliated with universities. They have rarely studied private hospitals because it is difficult to

141

gain entrance to them, even for research purposes. The head nurse at the private hospital where I gathered data said that the patients were paying to insure their privacy; research would make this privacy problematic. The majority of patients admitted to state hospitals are diagnosed as being schizophrenic. The proportion of cases of depression at private hospitals is much greater, and patients seen as private outpatients, a group almost never studied, are even more likely to be depressed.[11]

THEORETICAL EXPLANATIONS FOR DEPRESSION

There are three major theoretical explanations of depression (the biochemical and learning theory approaches will not be discussed). Psychiatrists distinguish between misfortune and depression. But what is a misfortune but a depression that "significant others"—relatives, friends, colleagues, doctors—consider an "appropriate response?" Thus, depression is a culture-bound and class-bound term. The first is the classic Freudian position which relates depression to the internalization of an ambivalently-loved person who has been lost. The individual who has lost the person then turns the hostility he felt towards him against himself.[20] The second, the ego-psychological approach, based on Freud's later writings, sees depression as a conflict within the ego itself.[7] Depression results when the ego is unable to live up to its goals. The third, an existential approach, considers depression the state that results when the individual finds that his world is meaningless.[6] None of these approaches is completely contradictory. They all assume that depression is the result of loss; loss of an ambivalently loved person in the first case, loss of goal in the second case, and loss of meaning in the third.

There is actually little empirical evidence for any of these conceptualizations. The evidence for the Freudian position concerning aggression is as follows: Clinical data showing that individuals suffering from depression whose "presented self" is unaggressive, have tremendous amounts of hostility which they are able to express during the process of psychotherapy;[12] Eaton and Weil's[16] study of the Hutterites which showed that in a group where depression is the most common form of emotional illness, aggression is tabooed; and finally the higher rate of depression for women,[41] if one is willing to accept the assumption that women are less likely than men to express aggression.

Major support for Bibring's ego-psychological theory of depression comes from clinical knowledge of individuals who have become depressed when they have not been able to reach their goals. Gerson and his associates[24] believe that Bibring's formulations are attractive because, among psychoanalytic theories, his most readily allow for hostility directed outward as well as inward during the onset of and during the recovery from severe depressive states.

There is a good deal of evidence supporting the existential assumption that man must have meaning in his life. Numerous psychological studies, stemming from the Gestalt tradition, such as Festinger's[18] theory of cognitive dissonance,

142

show that man must pattern his environment so that it "makes sense." Becker cites Field's[6] study of emotionally ill middle-aged women in Ghana as evidence supporting his position relating depression to a loss of meaning. Field,[19] an anthropologist and psychiatrist, discovered that many women, particularly at the onset of the involutional period of life, considered themselves witches and went to the shrines to be cured. These women may have suffered from role loss as well as loss of meaning, because among the Ackhan, one of the groups, the matrilineal kinship structure, which involved men visiting their wives only at night may have led to isolation at middle age for these women if their husbands stopped visiting them.[28] Becker[6] interprets the situation of the woman in this manner: "She raises large families with extreme care, is an excellent housekeeper and businesswoman as well. There is enough significant activity in her life to provide ample self-justification. But often the fruit of her labor is lavished by the husband on a younger bride, when the wife grows old . . . How is she to justify this utter subversion of life-meaning?" . . . Fortunately, the culture itself provides a ready rationalization. Verbalizations are ready-made with which to construct a framework of meaning and justification; the continuity of the staged drama of one's life experience need not be broken; the woman can simply acknowledge that *all along* she has been a witch. Thus the circle is closed: 'I have become useless because I have always been evil. I deserve this fate. I deserve to be hated' . . . The alternative to this—namely, the realization that perhaps *life has no meaning*—is much more difficult to come by" [pp. 116, 117].

Additional research on the subject has been done by Deykin and coworkers[49] and Brissett.[8] From the data Field presents, however, a Freudian interpretation cannot be ruled out. Becker's interpretation of the guilt of depressed women, an attempt to make the tragedies that have befallen them "make sense," is more parsimonious than is the classic Freudian explanation. The latter requires two assumptions: first, that the lost person has been hated as well as loved, and second, that the lost person has been internalized so that the guilt is, in fact, anger directed against the introjected person.

One possible way of combining the Freudian position concerning anger directed inward and the existential position concerning loss of meaning may be the following. People who are intrapunitive, who do not express their anger, especially if they are women, are conforming to the culture "norms." Since they have been "good," they expect to be rewarded. Therefore, when their husbands or children leave them, their world may no longer make sense. Thus, introjected anger leads to "proper" behavior which in turn leads to expectations of reward. When this reward does not materialize, but in fact tragedy strikes, they suffer from a loss of meaning and become depressed. This interpretation is also valid for other categories of depressed people. For example, involutional depression was found among the old socialist pioneers, the original founders of the Israeli kibbutzim, when they felt that their life patterns, the hardships they had endured, had come to nought because Israel was becoming another bourgeois nation-state.[34]

143

Briefly then, all the theories presented view depression as a response to a loss. The loss of a person, however, as described in the traditional Freudian approach, or the loss of a goal or an ideal, as described in the ego-psychological approach, may result in a loss of meaning for the individual. For neither Becker, the existentialist, nor Bibring, the ego-psychologist, does the feeling toward the lost object (goal, ideal, person, meaning) need to have been ambivalent. Therefore, while the *cause* of the depression may be conceptualized differently, the situation the individual finds himself in need not differ. The concept presented below to account for depression among middle-aged women, namely maternal role loss, is consistent with all of these approaches since it refers to loss. While it is unnecessary to assume that the lost child has been ambivalently loved, this is certainly possible. It is assumed, however, that the mother-child role of a mother who is over-involved in the maternal role is the major factor giving meaning to her life.

A SOCIOLOGICAL APPROACH TO DEPRESSION

Let us now present a sociological approach to depression. Role theory furnishes a mechanism to account for the manner in which social structural factors affect the individual; it conceptualizes the link between the society and the person. The two most common approaches to the role in American sociology stem from the writings of Linton and Mead. The Linton[30] approach accounts for stability in role behavior over a period of time and is essentially deterministic in nature. Roles are external and constraining.[25] Because roles are learned as part of the socialization process, it follows that different subcultures, such as different ethnic groups, should have different roles, norms, and expectations. Dahrendorf[13] notes that Durkheim "comes close to the category of role" when he states, in *Rules of the Sociological Method,*[15] when defining "social facts": "I fulfill my obligations as brother, husband, or citizen, if I honor my contracts, perform duties that are defined without reference to myself and my actions in law and custom. Even if these duties are in accord with my own sentiments and I feel subjectively their reality, such reality is objective, for I have not created it; I have merely inherited it as a result of my education." The view of the role of women, particularly the Jewish mother phenomenon which is described later in the chapter, can be thought of in Lintonian terms. This role, which is structurally conducive to depression, is learned during childhood socialization and is reinforced by the institutions of society.

The relevant part of symbolic interactionist theory, derived from the work of Mead, is its conceptualization of the interrelationship that exists between the role and the self. One's concept of self stems from one's roles; thus, a loss of a role relationship and a loss of significant others, can result in a sense of "mutilated self." This phrase is used by Rose[37] when he discussed involutional psychosis, a diagnostic term for depression appearing for the first time in middle age, somewhat later in men than in women. It is significant that although the term involutional implies a physiological referent, the times of appearance coincide with the loss of identity-giving roles for both sexes—the maternal role for the woman and the work role for the man.

The conception of self is actually a view of how one relates to major significant others whose roles are determined by the social structure. Since one's conception of self is learned by the selective identification of certain roles which appear to be the most congruent, self-esteem stems from a sense of adequacy in the most salient roles. Because the most important roles for women in our society are those of wife and mother, one might predict that the loss of either of these roles could result in a loss of self-esteem—resulting in the feeling of worthlessness and uselessness that characterizes most depression. For example, one woman said to me:

> I don't feel like I'm wanted. I don't feel at all that I'm wanted. I just feel like nothing, I don't feel anybody cares, and nobody's interested, and they don't care whether I do feel good or I don't feel good. I'm pretty useless . . . I feel like I want somebody to feel for me but nobody does.

Since a feeling of well-being is dependent on a positive conception of self, it is dependent on the roles available to the individual. When people are given the "Who am I" test to get at their self-concept, they almost always respond in terms of their various roles—wife, mother, lawyer, daughter, and so forth. Women whose identity is derived mainly from their role as mothers rather than as wives, whose significant others are limited to their children, are in a difficult situation when their children leave home and former patterns of social interaction between them are disrupted. These women's self-conceptualizations must change, however, some have personalities too rigid to enable them to make this change. They are overcommitted to the maternal role and then, in middle age, suffer the unintended consequences of this commitment. Men whose primary identity comes from their occupation would have similar problems on retirement. For example, some retired professional soldiers suffer from involutional psychosis.[26]

There recently has been an upsurge of interest in depression, largely manifested in studies on animals, particularly the results of maternal separation on young primates,[27, 32] on pharmacology, concerning the effectiveness of drugs in treating depression, and on genetic factors, particularly in manic-depressive, or bipolar subjects.[9, 22] The *Diagnostic and Statistical Manual II* (1968) has changed the classification of depression making "involutional psychotic reaction" a subcategory of "major affective disorders," while "involutional paranoid state" is now listed with paranoid states. "Psychotic depressive reaction" is now in a separate category.[42] Beck has called attention to the cognitive style of individuals who are suffering from depression which includes a pessimistic view, a negative self-image, a view of the future as more of the present, holding continual hardship, frustration, and deprivation.[4, 5] Gaylin[23] states that since the depressed individual's sense of self-esteem is regulated by external supplies, if his narcissistic needs are not satisfied, his level of self-esteem diminishes dangerously. Seligman and associates,[39,40] using learning theory and experimenting with dogs, found the animals gave up and passively accepted electric shock because in earlier trials they were helpless to avoid it. Seligman[39] believes there are significant parallels between learned helplessness in dogs and depression in humans[39] and suggests that individuals be given experiences with mastery to prevent depression. In addition, an interdisciplinary group at Yale University has been studying depression, particularly depressed women, for a number of years. Their work is noteworthy for the presence of a "normal" control group, and they have been investigating the life stresses and roles and their relation to depression.[36,44]

Depression as a Symptom Choice

The problem of symptom choice is still puzzling for the behavioral sciences. One sociocultural factor relevant to symptom choice is the characteristic mode of adapting to stress in a given subculture or family. Thus, if the individual sees his significant others adapting to stress by drinking, or withdrawing, or taking drugs, then this may be incorporated into his repertoire of behavior. Similarly, depression may be learned as the appropriate behavioral response to difficult situations.

But depression has special significance when it is present in individuals who are experiencing a role loss, particularly a loss of a spouse or child. Depression affords the individual secondary gains such as sympathy and attention from her or his family and the ability to control them subtly by manipulating their guilt feelings. Through these mechanisms, the depressed woman may regain what was lost when her children grew away from her. She could not receive this increased sympathy were she to respond to stress by resorting to acting-out behavior such as promiscuity or alcoholism. It is not suggested, however, that this choice is conscious.

This theory was tested in a study of depressed middle-aged women. Such data are important for several reasons. First, as previously mentioned, depression has not been studied by sociologists. Second, the middle age stage in the life cycle has been an area relatively ignored in social research. This stage is important from a practical viewpoint because, with the drop in maternal death rate and the increased use of contraceptives resulting in fewer children, more women are likely to reach the postparental stage of the family life cycle while in middle age. Third, knowledge of the interactive patterns, values and attitudes of middle-aged women can add to the sociological knowledge about role changes. It is at this stage in the life cycle that women tend to lose certain roles and gain others; some roles expand and others contract. Fourth, there is contradictory evidence in theory as to whether middle age *is* a problem for women. By attempting to specify the conditions under which middle-aged women become depressed, this study which I call "Portnoy's Mother's Complaint" offers an explanation for these contradictory theories and beliefs. The clinical literature, the data on hospitalization for mental illness, and the Stirling County studies show that middle age is a particularly stressful period for women. Some empirical studies have shown, however, that most women do not find this stage difficult.

ROLE LOSS IN DEPRESSION

I have hypothesized that the departure of the children would be more stressful for women whose primary role was that of a mother rather than that of a wife or of a career woman. In the traditional Jewish family, the main role for the woman is that of a mother. Thus, the difference between the two approaches to middle age may be a result of clinicians making generalizations about a population that is more susceptible to the stresses of middle age—the Jewish mother.[45, 46]

From the theoretical position previously discussed, I derived a number of hypotheses which I will summarize. (1) Depressed women would be more likely to experience a role loss than would nondepressed women. (2) There would be a higher proportion of depressed than of nondepressed women with maternal role loss. The effect of compensating factors and aggravating factors was predicted. (3) Certain roles would be structurally conducive to increasing the effect of the loss of other roles. (4) Impending role loss would also be associated with depression. (5) Depression among middle-aged women with maternal role loss would be related to the family structure and typical interactive patterns of the ethnic group to which they belong. Particular attention was given to the Jewish family to provide a test of the hypothesis concerning overprotective and overinvolved relationships with children. Preliminary statements regarding other ethnic groups were made for comparative purposes.[3, 50]

Because depression in middle age is sometimes attributed to the hormonal changes during menopause, I first conducted a cross-cultural study of 30 societies using the Human Relations Area Files. In addition, I studied six cultures intensively. An analysis of all these cultures showed that societies *had* roles available for postmenopausal women, that frequently the woman's status rose at this life-cycle stage, that the two societies in which woman's status decreased were similar to ours, and that, since in most societies middle age was not usually considered an especially stressful period for women, explanations of such stress based on biological changes of the menopause must be rejected.[2]

Next, the records of 533 women who had no previous record of hospitalization for mental illness, who were between the ages of 40 and 59, and whose final diagnosis was functional rather than organic, were examined and abstracted using *five* mental hospitals in the Los Angeles area. The use of five hospitals had three advantages. First, since three of the hospitals were relatively nonstigmatic, the sample included women who would not have entered a state hospital; second, the large and heterogeneous sample obtained made possible the introduction of controls for both ethnicity and social status; third, the results could not merely be a function of *one* hospital's diagnostic style or philosophy.

In addition to the cross-cultural and the epidemiological studies, I conducted a total of 20 intensive interviews at two hospitals to obtain information that was unavailable from the patients' records, to give the women questionnaires used in studies with "normal" middle-aged women, and to give them the projective biography test—a test consisting of 16 pictures showing women at different stages in their life cycle and in different roles.

I will now define certain terms that were employed in the studies. First, role loss: it could be either partial or complete. Maternal role loss meant at least one child was not living at home. Marital role loss meant that the woman was widowed, divorced, or separated. Occupational role loss meant that the women had become unemployed prior to the onset of symptoms. Overprotective or overinvolved relationships with children were coded when a statement such as "my whole life was my husband and my daughter" was found on the record, or if, for example, the patient entered the hospital following the child's engagement or marriage. Ratings of role loss, relationships with children and husband were made "blind," that is, from a history which omitted references to symptomatology, ethnicity, or diagnosis.

Middle age was considered to be the years between 40 and 59. Originally 65 was planned as the upper limit, but it was feared that organic brain damage would contaminate diagnoses at that age. Fortunately, a few women over 60 were interviewed and from them I learned the stress of the loss of the grandmother role—when grandchildren they previously baby-sat for became adolescent and the grandmothers were no longer wanted.

Five methods were used to overcome diagnostic biases. First, the sample was drawn from *five* hospitals, so that the results could not be caused by the diagnostic policies or philosophy at one hospital. Second, those with neurotic depressive illness were merged with women with involutional, psychotic, and manic depressive illnesses, since it was suspected that patients who would be diagnosed as being "neurotic depressed" at an upper-class hospital would be diagnosed as being "involutional depressed" at a lower-middle class hospital. This suspicion was borne out. Even people who are skeptical about diagnoses will agree that, in general, there is a difference between those with depressive illnesses and those suffering from schizophrenia (the second largest diagnostic category in the sample). Third, a symptom check list was used in the analysis of data, and it was found that patients diagnosed as being depressed differed significantly from those given other diagnoses for almost all the symptoms.

Fourth, a case history of a woman who had exhibited the symptoms of both depressive and paranoid illness was distributed to the psychiatric residents at the teaching hospital for blind diagnosis. In half the cases the woman was called Jewish and in the other half Presbyterian. The results showed no difference in number of stigmatic diagnoses between the Jews and Presbyterians since both the most and least number of stigmatic diagnoses were given to Presbyterians. Fifth, 39 Minnesota Multiphasic Personality Inventory profiles of the women from one hospital sample were obtained and given to a psychologist to diagnose blind. He rated them on an impairment continuum. The results supported the decision to combine those with psychotic, involutional, and neurotic depressive illnesses because the ratio of mild and moderate to serious and very serious was the same for all these groups. But all those with a diagnosis of schizophrenia were rated serious or very serious.

Women with diagnoses of depression were compared with those with other diagnoses. This paper will focus on those with maternal role loss. While marital role loss was also associated with depression, and the interviews indicated it resulted in a negative self-image and a normless state, it can occur anytime during the life cycle, while the loss of the maternal role is most characteristic of middle-aged women.

The data indicate that depression is increasingly associated with the following states: women with role loss, maternal role loss, housewives with maternal role loss, middle-class housewives with maternal role loss, women with maternal role loss having overprotective or overinvolved relationships with their children, and housewives with maternal role loss who have overprotective or overinvolved relationships with their children. Depression was also associated with *impending* role loss, that is, if a child were about to marry or go away or a husband were going to obtain a divorce. The *symptom* of depression was associated with maternal but not with other forms of role loss. That is, women who had symptoms of depressive illness but who were not diagnosed as being depressed were likely to have experienced maternal role loss.

The Influence of Ethnicity

Ethnicity was the most important factor associated with depression. Jews exhibited high, Blacks low, and those of Anglo-Saxon ancestry intermediate rates. There were too few Orientals and women with Spanish surnames to analyze. Evidence for depression as a behavior pattern resulting from traditional Jewish socialization was supported by the finding that Jewish women whose mothers were born in this country had a rate of depression midway between that of Jewish women with European mothers and that of women of Anglo-Saxon parentage. While 84 per cent of the 122 Jewish patients were diagnosed as being depressed, only 47 per cent of the non-Jewish women were so diagnosed. But when only women who had overprotective or overinvolved relationships with their children with maternal role loss were compared, the difference between Jews and non-Jews was reduced to 11 per cent. So, although Jewish women were more likely to have had this pattern of interaction with their children, when non-Jewish women had established such a pattern, they too were likely to respond to maternal role loss with depression.

The low rate of depression found among Black middle-aged women was predicted on the basis of the family structure, where the mother often cares for her grandchildren while her daughter works. If she does not live with her adult child, because of the constraints of segregated housing she is more likely to live near her children than is her White counterpart. Thus, she would be less likely to feel the loss of the maternal role. We have no way of knowing, from a hospitalized sample, about the prevalence of depressed Black women. Since individuals suffering from depression are not likely to come to the attention of the police unless they attempt suicide, and since psychiatric vocabularies of explanation are not as common in groups with little education and/or rural origin,[2] it is possible that there are significant numbers of depressed middle-aged Black women who have not been taken notice of. This failure to hospitalize for depression would probably not be as common among the other groups in the sample.

Psychodynamically, depression is considered the internalization of aggression. Several results I obtained supported this contention. For example, women married for the first time had a higher rate of depression than women who were divorced or remarried. In order for a woman to seek a divorce she must assume that her partner is at fault. An intrapunitive person of course would blame herself. This does not take into consideration that some of the husbands may have asked for the divorce. Of the 16 pictures shown to the women interviewed, the picture portraying an angry woman was the one liked *least* by most of the women. Other data collected suggested that these women did not admit or were not aware of their angry feelings. For example, one woman who had devoted 12 years to caring for her hyperactive, brain-damaged son, and who became depressed after he had to be placed in an institution, said: "It was extremely hard on me, and I think it has come out now. Very hard. I never knew I had the amount of patience. That child never heard a raised voice."

I had originally assumed that the depression surrounding the departure of children could be buffered if the woman became involved with an occupation in which she had intrinsic interest. I believed that a meaningful occupational role could be expanded to fill the gap. Considering I was a graduate student in the womb of the university at that time, perhaps I can be excused for my naivete. The data did not show that women with such roles were able to use them as meaningful alternatives. I thought it was because so few of the women were "higher professionals"—physicians, lawyers, or professors. Rather, they were nurses and school teachers. From the interview material, it had also been apparent that the one woman of the twenty who was a nurse was not greatly involved in her profession. Far from considering it a calling, she had become a nurse only when she needed the money, and had stopped working when she was married. The norms of our society are such that a woman is not *expected* to fulfill herself through an occupation, but rather through the traditional feminine roles of wife and mother. More than that, she is not *allowed* to do so. The great discrimination against "uppity women"—women professionals, the cruel humor, not being taken seriously, the lower pay scale, the invisibility both literally and metaphorically, make it almost suicidal for a woman to attempt to give meaning to her life through her work.

Some psychoanalytic explanations of menopausal depression, such as that of Helene Deutsch,[14] claim that it is the "masculine" women who become depressed

150

at this time. However, my data, including the attitudes expressed in the interviews, showed that it was the women who assumed the traditional feminine role—who were housewives, who stayed married to their husbands, who were not overtly aggressive, in short who adhered to the traditional norms, who responded with depression when their children left. Even the Minnesota Multiphasic Personality Inventory masculinity-femininity scores for the women at the one hospital where they were available were one-half a standard deviation *more* feminine than the mean. These findings are consistent with Cohen's[12] theory of depression which states that feelings of depression are most frequent among those who are "most cohesively identified with their families." Ernest Becker's theory of existential depression among middle-aged women is borne out because these martyr mothers thought that by being "good" ultimately they would be rewarded. When there was no pot of gold at the end of the rainbow, their life pattern seemed meaningless. As one woman said:

> I felt that I trusted and they took advantage of me. I'm very sincere, but I wasn't wise. I loved, and loved strongly and trusted, but I wasn't wise. I deserved something, but I thought, if I give to others they'll give to me. How could they be different, but you see those things hurted me very deeply and when I had to feel that I don't want to be alone, and I'm going to be alone, and my children will go their way and get married—of which I'm wishing for and then I'll still be alone and I got more and more alone, and more and more alone.

The interviews covered the skeleton of statistics with the flesh of individual lives. The time sequence and the importance of the stresses these women faced, their attitudes, values, interactive patterns with me as well as with their children, and their life styles emerged. Unfortunately, during the five-month period I was interviewing, only one nondepressed middle-aged woman was admitted to one of the two hospitals I used for the purpose, so woman with depressive illnesses could not be compared with those of a nondepressive category.

Only a few findings will be reported. First, any doubts about the validity of the inferences from the hospital charts that the women were overprotective, martyrs, and conventional were dispelled. Although she was a patient and I was an interviewer and a stranger, one Jewish woman forced me to eat candy, saying, "Don't say no to me." Another gave me unsolicited advice on whether I should remarry and to whom, and a third said she would make a party for me when she left the hospital. Another example of the extreme nurturant patterns was shown by a fourth who insisted on caring for another patient who had just returned from a shock treatment while I was interviewing her. She also attempted to find other women for me to interview. The vocabulary of motives invoked by the Jewish women generally attributed their illness to their children. They complained about not seeing their children often enough. The non-Jewish women were more restrained and said they wanted their children to be independent. Two of the Jewish women had lived with their children, wanted to live with them again, and their illness was precipitated when their children forced them to live alone. However, living with their children was not a satisfactory arrangement for the women in the sample, since the few women having this arrangement were all depressed. For example, one woman complained:

Why is my daughter so cold to me? Why does she exclude me? She turns to her husband . . . and leaves me out. I don't tell her what to do, but I like to feel my thoughts are wanted.

A dramatic expression of the traditional Jewish family structure as described in *Life Is With People*[46] was one woman's statement, "My son is my husband and my husband is my son." All the women with children, when asked what they were most proud of, stated "my children." Occasionally, after this, they mentioned their husbands.

The conventionality and the rigidity of the women interviewed were shown by their ranking of seven roles available to middle-aged women: being a homemaker; taking part in church, club, and community activities; companion to husband; helping parents; sexual partner; paying job; helping children. In middle age it is necessary to be flexible so that new roles can be assumed. But the women most frequently ranked "helping my children" first or second, although only one of the seven women whose children were all living at home ranked it first, and one ranked it second. Since it is difficult to help children who are no longer living at home, women who value this behavior more than any other are in a difficult situation. They are frustrated in their attempts to behave in the way that is most important to them. Items that were not chosen are as interesting to note as items that were; "helping my parents" was ranked first by only one woman. Her hospitalization had followed her mother's move to Chicago after she had remodeled her apartment so that her mother could live with her. This furnishes another example of a woman whose major value, her most salient role, has been frustrated. No woman listed "being a sexual partner to my husband" first, and only one woman listed it second. Three married women did not include it in their ranking, indicating the lack of importance or rejection of this role. It is apparent that although eight of the women worked outside the home, the occupation role was not important to them. Three did not even list it. Most dramatic was one woman who simply listed "helping my children" and put down no other roles.

In short, it appears as if it is precisely those roles that the women view as important, the roles of homemaker and mother, that become constricted as the women age. Conversely, the roles that could be expanded at this time, the sexual partner role, the occupational role, and the organizational role (taking part in church, club, and community activities) are not important to these women.

The women interviewed were given the Projective Biography Test—16 pictures showing women in different roles and at different stages in their life cycle. The clinical psychologist who devised the test analyzed the protocols without knowing my hypotheses. He considered their responses support for the

152

hypothesis because so many of the women were, as he said, "complete mothers," showing total identification with the maternal role. I analyzed the content of responses to the sexy, the pregnancy, the old age, and the angry pictures. Because of space limitations I will present only the response to the old age picture. This picture showed an old woman sitting in a rocking chair in front of a fireplace. To the extent that projective tests may be valid, the nine women who did not include this picture in their stories of a woman's life hold negative attitudes toward aging. Only one woman used the picture in the story and responded positively to it. Two used it, but denied the aging aspects of it. An example of such denial is the following response: "Here she is over here sitting in front of the fireplace, and she's got her figure back, and I suppose the baby's gone off to sleep and she's relaxing." This woman, however, interpreted every picture with reference to a baby.

Six expressed negative attitudes toward the picture, two responses were uncodeable. One woman who used the picture in the story said, "And this scene I can't stand. Just sitting alone in old age there by some fireplace all by herself (pause) turning into something like that. And to me this is too lonely. A person has to slow down sometime and just sit, but I would rather be active, and even if it would be elderly I wouldn't want to live so long that I wouldn't have anything else in life but to just sit alone and you know, just in a rocking chair." She is a woman who does not want to "disengage" in old age. Another woman who was divorced and had both her children away from home said, "This could look very much like me. I'm sitting, dreaming, feeling so blue." When she chose that as the picture not liked, she said, "Least of all I don't like this one at all. That's too much like I was doing. Sitting and worrying and thinking and . . ."

In the inquiry period, one more gave a positive response, four gave a negative response, and one response was uncodeable. One woman who was divorced and living alone did not use the picture in her story. After listing eight other pictures which were like her life, she said, "I don't like to point to that one." One person liked this picture best, but did not perceive the woman as old, while six women included this picture among the ones they liked least. These indicate that the women interviewed do not look forward to old age. This response may not be statistically deviant. However, these women were facing old age, and their rejection of this stage, whether or not such rejection is normal was a source of stress. In addition, since these women appear to be energetic, the inactivity of old age may be seen by them as particularly being stressful.

At this point, I would like to briefly comment on the relationship that exists between defense mechanisms and the life cycle. Withdrawal as a defense in a society valuing instrumental activism is likely to cause problems early in life. However, if one uses being active as a defense mechanism, one can manage very well in our society, barring physical illness, until retirement for men or the departure of children for women. The interview data, and certain comments on the hospital charts, for example, "She needed to keep busy all the time," indicated that many of the women had such systems of defense. This mechanism had been

153

rewarded by the society at earlier stages in the women's life cycle. However, later, when many women were physically ill, and there was little for them to do, this life style was no longer effective.

Because of the limitations imposed by a study based on a hospitalized sample, a prevalence study *should* be conducted. Undoubtedly, there are many depressed middle-aged women who are not in mental hospitals. Those women of higher socioeconomic status, particularly those with college education, who have psychiatric vocabularies, may be in treatment with private psychotherapists. Those women with less education, who do not think in psychiatric terms, may be doing nothing about their depression *per se,* although they may be possibly treating the physiological symptoms that accompany the depression. Until such a survey is completed, knowledge of the relationship between role loss and depression must be limited.

However, it does seem clear that when women are socialized into traditional female roles, deriving their conceptions of self solely from the mother and wife roles without any true sense of identity coming from themselves rather than vicariously from the accomplishments of their husbands and children, they are prone to depression in middle age if they lose these roles. Recent changes in our society such as the increasing participation of women in the labor force and the growth of the women's liberation movement which gives emotional support to women deviating from traditional roles, should reduce the incidence of depression among middle-aged women in the future.

Such changes are particularly important because recent analyses of census data[38] show that "maternity has become a very small part of the adult woman's life." For a woman who marries a man two years older when she is 22, who has two children two years apart, and who dies at 74, "only 12 per cent of her life will be spent in full-time maternal care of preschool-age children, 23 per cent of her adult life will be spent without a husband, and 41 per cent of her adult life will be spent with a husband but no children under 18."

There is pain in living—physical and psychic. Much of it is existential, or inherent in the conditions of our existence. But some of it stems from particular social structural and institutional arrangements which generate feelings of helplessness, being unwanted and feeling unloved. In short, there are patterns in our society conditions, and constraints which lead to lowered levels of self-esteem among individuals—this leads to depression.

As Gaylin[23] says in his epilogue to *The Meaning of Despair:*

To the extent that one's sense of well-being, safety, or security is dependent on love, money, social position, power, drugs, or obsessional defenses—to that extent one will be threatened by its loss. When the reliance is preponderant, the individual despairs of survival and gives up. It is that despair which has been called depression. [It occurs] When the adult gives up hope in his ability to cope and sees himself incapable of either fleeing or fighting [pp. 390, 391].

In a more sociological vein, Myers and his associates[48] state:

> The finding that the exit of an individual from the immediate social field of the respondent is associated more strongly with impairment than comparable entrance emphasizes the importance of object loss in psychopathology in our culture, and suggests that there is a hierarchy of role transformations with respect to psychiatric symptomatology. American society with its secular nontraditional attitudes has left the individual somewhat alone to cope with loss. Grief and mourning are denied to a larger extent in our society than in many others. Although we do have rituals to help the individual endure a loss, much of this is in the form of denial. With a pervasive skepticism of a world to come, once a loss occurs, it is permanent and probably quite shattering to the individual. Ours is a society bent upon the pursuit of 'happiness,' and . . . more meaningful systems of social and interpersonal support probably have developed around gain than around loss [p. 156].

Such a position supports the point made in the first section of this paper about the illegitimacy of feelings of depression, and the concept of metadepression—being depressed because you are feeling depressed.

Cannot patterns of socialization be developed that would reduce dependency needs patterns where the concept of self rather than that of others is the major reinforcing agent? In traditional Jewish socialization, guilt is the means of social control, eating or not eating symbolizes acceptance or rejection of the person offering the food (usually the mother), and aggression is taboo. Since those who are depressed often feel guilty, they frequently turn their anger (aggression) against themselves and eat little, it is obvious how such socialization facilitates depression as a response to stress. Additionally, depression stems from a feeling of helplessness. There is a long sociological tradition of studying alienation and its effects. The most important (and the Marxian) meaning of alienation is powerlessness, so the helplessness of those with depressive illnesses can be considered alienation. By giving "power to the people," by creating a means whereby individuals have more control over their lives, we can attempt to reduce the helpless state in which too many people find themselves.

It is too easy to focus on the secondary gain depression brings, or, as sociologists, to look at statistics, forgetting the exquisite agony of each individual who makes up the statistics. As sociologists and as human beings, it is our responsibility to point out the depression inducing features of our social structure, as I attempted to do when I discussed the traditional female role. And, in addition to noting these roles, values, norms, contradictions, and conflicts, both interpersonal and global, we should use our sociological imaginations to change the society so as to reduce the tragedy of meaningless suffering. For, as Gaylin[23] says, "It is part of the wonder of man that even the state of hopelessness can be used to generate hope" [p. 391].

REFERENCES

1. BART, P.: Depression in Middle Aged Women: Some Sociocultural Factors. Unpublished dissertation, UCLA. Ann Arbor, Michigan: University Microfilms, 1967.
2. BART, P.: "Why Woman's Status Changes in Middle Age." *Sociological Symposium* 3: 1-18, 1969.
3. BART, P.: Mother Portnoy's Complaint. *Trans-Action* 8: 69-74, 1970.
4. BECK, A. T.: *Depression: Clinical, Experimental and Theoretical Aspects.* New York: Hoeber Medical Division, Harper and Row, 1967.
5. BECK, A. T.: "The Core Problem in Depression: The Cognitive Triad." *Science and Psychoanalysis* 17:47-55, 1970.
6. BECKER, E.: *The Revolution in Psychiatry.* Glencoe, Illinois: The Free Press, 1964.
7. BIBRING, E.: "The Mechanism of Depression," in Phyllis Greenacre (ed.): *Affective Disorders.* New York: International Universities Press, 1953, Pp. 13-48.
8. BRISSETT, D. D.: Clinical Depression: A Sociological Inquiry. Unpublished dissertation. Ann Arbor, Michigan: University Microfilms, 1968.
9. BRODIE, H., KEITH, H., AND LEFF, M. J.: Bipolar Depression: A Comparative Study of Patient Characteristics. Paper presented at the American Psychiatric Association meeting, San Francisco, May, 1970.
10. BURTON, R.: *The Anatomy of Melancholy.* New York: Tudor Publications. (trans.), 1968.
11. CANNON, M. S., AND REDICK, R. W.: Differential Utilization of Psychiatric Facilities by Men and Women United States 1970. Rockville, Maryland: Department of Health, Education, and Welfare Publication No. (HSM) 73-9005, 1973.
12. COHEN, Y. A.: The Sociological Relevance of Schizophrenia and Depression, in Yehudi A. Cohen (ed.): *Social Structure and Personality.* New York: Holt, Rinehart and Winston, 1961, Pp. 477-485.
13. DAHRENDORF, R.: *Homo Sociologicus: The Theory of Society.* Stanford: Stanford University Press, 1968.
14. DEUTSCH, H.: *The Psychology of Women: A Psychoanalytic Interpretation, II.* New York: Grune and Stratton, 1945.
15. DURKHEIM, E.: *The Rules of the Sociological Method.* Glencoe, Illinois: The Free Press, 1956.
16. EATON, J. W., AND WEIL, R. J.: *Culture and Mental Disorders.* Glencoe, Illinois: The Free Press, 1955.
17. FARIS, R. E. L., AND DUNHAM, W. H.: *Mental Disorders in Urban Areas.* Chicago: The University of Chicago Press, 1939.
18. FESTINGER, L.: *A Theory of Cognitive Dissonance.* Evanston, Illinois: Row, Peterson, 1957.
19. FIELD, M. J.: *Search for Security.* Evanston, Illinois: Northwestern University Press, 1960.
20. FREUD, S.: Mourning and Melancholia, in James Strachey (ed.): *Collected Papers,* 5. London: The Hogarth Press, 1956, Pp. 152-169.
21. FRIEDAN, B.: *The Feminine Mystique.* New York: W. W. Norton and Company, 1963.
22. FULLER, J. L.: Genetics and Vulnerability to Experiental Deprivation. Paper presented at meeting of American Association for the Advancement of Science, Chicago, 1970.
23. GAYLIN, W. (ed.): *The Meaning of Despair: Psychoanalytic Contributions to Understanding Depression.* New York: Science House, Inc., 1968.
24. GERSON, E. S., CROMER, M., AND KLERMAN, G. L.: Hostility and Depression, *Psychiatry* 68:224-35, 1968.
25. GOFFMAN, E.: *Encounters.* Indianapolis: Bobbs-Merrill, 1961.
26. JACOBSEN, O.: Personal communication, 1963.
27. KAUFMAN, I. C.: Mother-Infant Separation in Monkeys: An Experimental Model. Paper presented to meeting of Animal Behavior Society, cosponsored by American Association for the Advancement of Science and the American Psychiatric Association, Chicago (December), 1970.
28. KUPER, H.: Personal communication, 1966.
29. LINSKY, A. S.: Community Structure and Depressive Disorders. *Social Problems* 17:121-131, 1969.
30. LINTON, R.: *The Cultural Background of Personality.* New York: Appleton-Century-Crofts, Inc., 1945.
31. MANDEL, A.: Personal communication, 1967.

32. McKINNEY, W. T., JR., SUOMI, S. J., AND HARLOW, H. F.: New Models of Separation with Depression in Rhesus Monkeys. Paper presented at the meeting of the American Association for the Advancement of Science (December), 1970.

33. MERTON, R.: Social Structure and Anomie, in *Social Theory and Social Structure*. Glencoe, Illinois: The Free Press, 1957, Pp. 131-160.

34. MOSES, R., AND KLEIGLER, D. S.: A Comparative Analysis of Institutionalization of Mental Health Values: The United States and Israel. Unpublished manuscript presented at the American Psychiatric Association meetings, New York, 1965.

35. PARK, R. E.: The City: Suggestions for the Investigation of Human Behavior in the Urban Environment. *American Journal of Sociology* 20: 577-612, 1916.

36. PAYKEL, E. S., MYERS, J. K., DIENELT, M., KLERMAN, G., LINDENTHAL, J., AND PEPPER, M. P.: Life Events and Depression, *Archives of General Psychiatry* 21 (6): 753-60, 1969.

37. ROSE, A.: A Socio-Psychological Theory of Neurosis, in Arnold Rose (ed.): *Human Behavior and Social Processes*. Boston: Houghton-Mifflin Company, 1962, Pp. 537-549.

38. ROSSI, A. S.: Family Development in a Changing World. *American Journal of Psychiatry* 128: 1057-1066, 1972.

39. SELIGMAN, M. E. P.: Fall into Helplessness. *Psychology Today* 7: 43-48, 1973.

40. SELIGMAN, M. E. P., MAIER, S. F., AND GEER, J. H.: Alleviation of Learned Helplessness in the Dog. *Journal of Abnormal Psychology* 73: 256-262, 1968.

41. SILVERMAN, C.: *Epidemiology of Depression*. Johns Hopkins, 1968.

42. SPITZER, R. L., AND WILSON, P. R.: A Guide to the New Nomenclature. *American Journal of Psychiatry* 124: 1619-1629, 1968.

43. *Time* Magazine, The Command Generation. July 19, 1966.

44. WEISSMAN, M. J., PAYKEL, E. S., SEIGEL, R., AND KLERMAN, G. L.: The Social Role Performance of Depressed Women: Comparison with a Normal Group. *American Journal of Orthopsychiatry* 41:390-405, 1971.

45. WOLFENSTEIN, M.: Two Types of Jewish Mothers, in Marshall Sklare (ed.): *The Jews*. Glencoe, Illinois: The Free Press, 1958, Pp. 520-534.

46. ZBOROWSKI, M., AND HERZOG, E.: *Life is With People*. New York: Schoken Books, 1952.

47. NISBET, R: *The Sociological Tradition*. New York: Basic Books, 1966.

48. MYERS, J. K., LINDENTHAL, J. J., AND PEPPER, M. P.: "Life Events and Psychiatric Impairment." *Journal of Nervous and Mental Disease* 152: 149-157, 1971.

49. DEYKIN, E. Y., JACOBSON, S., KLERMAN, G., AND SOLLOMON, M.: "The Empty Nest: Psychosocial Aspects of Conflict Between Depressed Women and Their Grown Children." *American Journal of Psychiatry* 122: 1422-1426, 1966.

50. BART, P.: *Portnoy's Mother's Complaint*. Not yet published.

CHAPTER 8

Sociology and the Study of Suicide: Issues and Controversies

JAMES M. HENSLIN
AND JAMES D. CAMPBELL

When we trace sociology's history, we find that suicide has been of major interest to sociologists since the development of sociology as an independent academic discipline. The study of suicide was intricately tied up with the emergence of sociology as a new academic area: Durkheim utilized an examination of suicide in order to demonstrate his sociologistic proposition—that there is a social reality that is independent of individual realities—and his derivative position that the academic community needed an independent discipline. Not only was the study of suicide important in launching sociology as an independent discipline then, but suicide remains an area of continuing interest to sociologists today, with, for example, 160 articles and 10 books on suicide being abstracted in *Sociological Abstracts* for the period of 1953 to 1970.

In this chapter we examine the relationship between sociology and the study of suicide, giving an overview of the approaches and findings by sociologists in this area and delineating current issues and controversies surrounding the sociology of suicide. We first examine the classic study in sociology that deals with this subject, Durkheim's *Suicide*.

Following this, we deal with the need for criticism of the sociological study of suicide, the ecological fallacy, suicide statistics and rates, unicausality and multicausality in theoretical explanations of suicide, an overview of relevant theories, and the social meanings of suicide. We conclude with a brief statement concerning the current state of sociological knowledge of suicide.

DURKHEIM AND THE STUDY OF SUICIDE

It is not easy for a new discipline to emerge in academia. The existing disciplines have the intellectual world cut up into small empires, jealously guarding any encroachment on their claimed intellectual territories. For an independent discipline to develop, it is necessary to demonstrate that there is subject matter that is not being handled by any of the established disciplines or that, even though the established disciplines are dealing with the subject, a new approach or methodology is needed to do so adequately.

Such was the case in the 1890's when Emile Durkheim was completing his doctorate. Convinced that the current approaches to the study of social phenomena were inadequate and that a new discipline was needed, Durkheim wrote *The Division of Labor in Society.*[10] Completing this, he turned to the study of suicide and wrote *Suicide*[11] as a means by which he could further convince others that sociology was, indeed, a legitimate discipline. It is probable that the reason Durkheim chose the study of suicide for this purpose was because through it he was able to contradict the commonly held view that suicide was an intensely individual act.[8] His data indicated that there are social forces that regulate suicide rates; although suicide rates vary from country to country and from subgroup to subgroup within each country, they possess a regularity that is indicative of the effect of external causes on the individual.

Martin[28] has argued that Durkheim's major contributions in *Suicide* are his attempts to integrate social factors into a general theory, to exclude nonsocial factors as explanatory, and to eliminate the need for a variety of special *ad hoc* theories to account for differences among specific social groups, for example, religious, occupational, marital, and age groups. Martin also praises Durkheim's *Suicide* for providing a "wealth of data on comparative suicide rates," as being "a classic contribution of sociological methodology," and says that "the book's truly great contribution is as a theory building endeavor."

In *Suicide* Durkheim[11] develops three major propositions: the suicide rate varies inversely with the degree of integration of religious society, domestic society, and political society. He combines these into a general proposition: "Suicide varies inversely with the degree of integration of the social groups of which the individual is a part." In spite of his laudatory attempt to incorporate all suicide into general theory, the fact that Durkheim provides no operational definition of integration is problematic. Without such an operationalization, the theory is untestable and irrefutable. As we discuss below, an inadequate operationalization of integration has continued to be one of the major failings of sociologists doing suicide research.

Although *Suicide* has become a classic in sociology, and one of the paradigms on which students of sociology develop their basic assumptions, it has recently become the center of controversy. Douglas[8] claims that sociologists have not really understood the study. He argues that sociologists have misinterpreted *Suicide* because they do not share Durkheim's general frames of reference; because of this "many of the most important statements in *Suicide* mean something different today to most sociologists from what they meant to Durkheim and his contemporaries." This is primarily due, Douglas says, to our lack of familiarity with the sources that Durkheim used and, most importantly, to a form of thought in *Suicide* that differs fundamentally from our own.

The major thought-form in which Durkheim differs from most sociologists currently is that he is a realist rather than a nominalist. According to Douglas,[8] Durkheim is ordinarily thought to be a nominalist, drawing conclusions and generalizations from the particulars of data; closer examination, however, indicates him to be a philosophical realist, starting from the general and moving to the particulars. Although Durkheim laid great claim to a positivistic approach in his study of social phenomena, including that of suicide, and even though he paid considerable attention to statistical data, *he began with general ideas about society and suicide and interpreted the data to fit his preconceived theory.*[8,30]

It has not been generally recognized that Durkheim began his study of suicide with a preconceived theory, forcing his data to match his theory, or that he inserted common-sense experience that twisted the meaning of the data in such a way that his theory became almost irrefutable. Sociologists have tended to approach Durkheim wearing glasses tinted with admiration for one of the great founding fathers of *Sociologica Academia* and have ordinarily not looked too closely or critically at what he actually wrote.

One factor that may have prevented Durkheim from being viewed too critically is his own protestations in *Suicide* that he is taking a nominalistic approach.[11] For example:

. . . . the sociologist must take as the object of his research, groups of facts clearly circumscribed, capable of ready definition, with definite limits, and adhere strictly to them [p. 36].

Although many sociologists have uncritically accepted this claim, Douglas[8] especially singles out Gibbs and Martin[17] for being impressed by Durkheim's rhetoric without a close examination of his actual performance.

Regardless of who is correct in the controversy about the proper way to understand *Suicide,* Durkheim's work has been of major importance in influencing the thought of sociologists, not only regarding the study of suicide but also regarding the sociological approach to the study of social phenomena. For example, Durkheim argued that each society contains varying degrees of egoism, altruism, and anomie, and that a balance of these three is necessary for the welfare of the society. Unfortunately, he did not show the interrelationship between these three variables as cause for the suicide rate; instead, he related suicide rate only to anomie.[8] This imputed relationship has been so wholeheartedly accepted by sociologists that one sociologist has even asserted that the suicide rate can be taken as an indication of the degree of anomie in a society.[33]

The Need for Criticism

The sociological study of suicide needs thorough-going criticism. Much of the criticism that we have appears to merely be *pro forma,* done for the sake of appearance, for a presentation of front before the sociological cadre that the researcher imagines is looking over his shoulder—*pro forma* with the substance gone. The following is one of the best examples of such "criticism." In a review of Maris'[27] *Social Forces in Urban Suicide,* Kinsey[23] says that he has "reservations concerning the theoretical model and methodology" used by Maris. Immediately following this, he says that Maris' book is "an outstanding piece of work," is "clearly written," and "could become (a) classic(s) in the study of suicide." How, one might wonder, can this be? If one really has reservations concerning the theory and method, what is left? Unfortunately, sociologists of suicide appear to be blinded by their own erudition and loyalties to one another—so much so that they deny one another the edifying benefit of honest criticism, criticism that might turn repetitive and blind alley research into productive paths. Douglas[8] is the major exception to this pattern.

A good example of this failure of criticism in sociological suicidology is the work of Maris. Maris[27] begins his book with the bold and laudable assertion that one of the major purposes of his book is "putting Durkheim to bed." He even states his case so strongly that he says: "this book is dedicated to 'forgetting' Durkheim in order that sociology of suicide as a science may not be lost." Unfortunately, Maris forgets his dedicated purpose somewhere along the line and ends up frequently referring back to Durkheim, even making such statements as, "It appears that most of these findings can be fitted into Durkheim's general theory of suicide."[27] One might say, to continue his own analogy, that Maris appears only to go to bed with Durkheim instead of putting him to bed.

Maris is by no means the only sociologist who approaches Durkheim in this way. Labovitz,[24] for example, has recently felt the need of paying homage to Durkheim by following such well travelled paths as the following:

> Countries with quite different features may have approximately the same (suicide) rate. For example, the climate, soil composition, and characteristics of the terrain of Canada and Puerto Rico are vastly different, yet their 1960 suicide rates are nearly equal [p. 63].

We might say that Durkheim is indeed alive and well—in the hearts, minds, and writings of those sociologists who are doing research on suicide.

Suicide represents a relatively minor social problem when we compare it to such matters as crime and mental illness. Yet when we examine the body of the sociological literature, we readily see that suicide has received a considerable amount of attention. It is possible that the accessibility of official suicide rates has been a main determinant of the broad sociological interests in the study of suicide. However, there are many areas of human life for which "official rates" are readily available. It appears to us that Durkheim has lent a sort of charismatic light to suicide research. It appears that sociology feels that it is legitimized through an emphasis on the positive, and sociologists traditionally feel that Durkheim blazed such a trail for sociology. As we have just indicated, there is another view of Durkheim's role, one that we hope is coming more to the forefront of contemporary American sociology. We hope that this paper is a contribution in that direction. In the following pages we shall attempt to present constructive criticisms of sociological research on suicide, with a sincere, though pessimistic, hope that this chapter will help sociologists move toward creative paths in suicide research, rather than merely following the well-trod, but unproductive, furrows of those who have gone before.

Ecological Fallacy in Sociology

From the ecological school of American sociology, those who wrote on suicide include Cavan,[4] Schmid,[36,38] and Zorbaugh.[40] Their approach to the study of suicide represents a moral position, and it can be briefly summarized as follows: as the effects of social values decrease, the suicide rate increases. Social disorganization is responsible for the decrease in the effect of social values and it is caused by mobility, anonymity, and the rate of contact with others, or the rate of social relations. Therefore, changes in the effect of social values can be considered instrumental in causing suicide.

The ecological approach has been described[34] as not being a theory but rather as an unsystematic, multifactored perspective in which the ecological theorists committed the *ecological fallacy;* that is, they assumed that ecological characteristics (for example, slum areas) are responsible for a man's behavior patterns (and even, for example, suicide). Although the general sociocultural system was considered to be the locus of causes of suicide, there was much confusion between *predisposing* factors (factors that determine the probability that certain individuals will commit suicide) and *precipitating* factors (factors that determine which individuals will commit suicide). The problem consisted of trying to explain why some individuals who share characteristics thought to be suicidogenic (for example, isolation) commit suicide, while others who have the same characteristic do not commit suicide. Why, in terms of their assumptions, does "social disorganization" produce "personal disorganization" in some individuals while it does not in others?

The ecological fallacy as it relates to suicide might be diagrammed as follows:

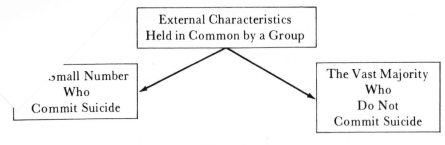

Figure 1

An example from criminology can further clarify the ecological fallacy. Is crime, as is sometimes thought, caused by ecological variables? If so, can knowledge of background variables provide the basis for predicting who will become a criminal, for example, parental income, education, type of housing, an individual's class standing in school, racial and ethnic characteristics, and number of siblings. Although we can fairly accurately predict the proportions of arrests for various crimes on the basis of knowledge of such background characteristics, we are not able to predict *who* will become a criminal. Certainly statisticians do not make such claims. If we approach our study of suicide or crime with the idea that background characteristics are causal variables, it is easy to end up committing the ecological fallacy. Rather than looking at ecological variables as causes of social action, attention must be focused on some intervening variable or defining process whereby those who are "predisposed" mediate relevant characteristics or events in such a way as to lead to a certain outcome, in this case, suicide and crime.

In trying to deal with this problem, some ecological theorists[4,13,36-38] began to emphasize the *social meanings* of ecological factors; that is, they noted that the same ecological characteristics do not have the same meaning for everyone, and individuals respond differentially to the same ecological factors on the basis of differing normative meanings. Promising as this strategy was, it was only an indication, and these theorists did not systematically pursue the relationship between individual and social meanings of ecological variables.[8]

THE USE OF OFFICIAL SUICIDE STATISTICS

A major criticism of sociological approaches to the study of suicide is that sociologists often develop hypotheses that are based on a particular operational definition of suicide, then check these hypotheses against official statistics with the assumption that the official statistics are compatible with their operational definitions. Douglas[8] forcefully makes the point that sociologists have paid only lip service to the possibility that their operational definitions and those of agents who gather suicide statistics do not match. He says that sociologists have not adequately checked out this presumed match but have instead worked on the assumption that it exists; thus, they are claiming confirmation or disconfirmation of hypotheses on only the flimsiest of evidence. It seems that most sociologists who use suicide statistics have gotten into such a rut that they cannot see anything but the furrow others have plowed before them. This furrow may not only be crooked but may even be in the wrong direction; nonetheless, sociologists appear willing to follow it for generations.

This uncritical use of official statistics by sociologists is based on two tacit assumptions: (1) officials make few errors in deciding whether a death is or is not by suicide, and (2) any errors they do make are "randomized," thus avoiding any systematic bias.[8] Accordingly, sociologists traditionally accept official suicide statistics as being reliable indicators of the suicide rate.

In order for a science to advance, it must clearly specify the meaning of the terms it uses. This is essential if findings from various studies are to be comparable. A major problem of contemporary sociology is a fundamental lack of comparability between the findings of various studies: researchers using the same concept operationalize it differently. This results in the chaotic state in which sociologists think that they are talking about the same thing when they are actually referring to entirely different, although sometimes related, phenomena. The myriad of laboratory studies in social psychology are especially marked by this fundamental deficiency. If, for example, the concept aggression or prejudice is operationalized in one study in one way but differently so in another, one is not certain but that the researchers are tapping two entirely different phenomena and that their measurements, although neat and perhaps even replicable, are actually measuring different things. Similar problems of comparability can be inadvertently created in survey research through changing the ordering or wording of key questions.

Although this problem is well recognized by sociologists in regard to laboratory studies and survey research, questions of validity are relatively rare when it comes to the official statistics in suicide research; they are not, however, entirely ignored. The issue was raised even prior to Durkheim, by de Guerry,[6] de Boismont,[3] and Legoyt.[25] Durkheim himself considered the matter and it has been raised by numerous subsequent researchers. But asking the question has been largely inconsequential. The validity issue typically has been dispensed with in a few sentences, with the researcher paying some sort of lip service to the problem, then stating something like, "Official statistics, although not perfect, are the best that we have available to us; therefore . . . ."[15]

The most extensive statement of the problem concerning the use of official suicide statistics has been made by Douglas.[8] He emphasized that the unreliability of official suicide statistics for developing and testing hypotheses is not an idle point, as some sociologists who blissfully continue their uncritical use of these data seem to suppose. As a case in point regarding the unreliability of official statistics, we can look at the category of "forcible rape" in the *Uniform*

Crime Reports. Here we find that of all forcible rapes reported to the police, 18 per cent are determined by police investigation to be unfounded. Additionally, all sorts of extraneous intersexual interaction gets included in this category that superficially appears to be unequivocal as to its contents. We find, for example, that a man might be arrested and charged with forcible rape for merely tickling a girl on her stomach and knees. We also find the following:

> The second case, not dissimilar, involved a man who inched near two young girls on a busy suburban street, then pinched one of them on the bottom. A police officer, who had been watching the encounter, immediately arrested the man. In his statement, the offender indicated that he frequently engaged in this sort of activity. His main satisfaction from it, he said, derived from frightening the girls. His case was also listed under the heading of forcible rape[5] [p. 182].

It is to the credit of Chappell and his associates that they did not uncritically accept the official classification of forcible rape, but, in making their comparative study of rapes in Los Angeles and Boston, they checked each police report in order to determine whether the same operational definitions were being followed by police officials in both cities. As a result of their critical approach to official statistics, they found the Boston police were using a different set of criteria than were the Los Angeles police, although the *Uniform Crime Reports* states in clear language the operational definition that is to be followed. Accordingly, to make their comparative study, Chappell and co-workers had to discard many of the cases from the Los Angeles arrest records.

The same validity problem holds true for suicide. Critical examination of coroners' records has led some researchers to question cases that are included as well as those that are excluded from the category "death by suicide." In my own research in this area, for example, I was surprised to find that the coroner sometimes includes as suicides cases of multiple gunshot wounds, while excluding cases that appeared to me to be suicides *prime facie.*

Durkheim[11] recognized that the official classification of *motives* for suicide was suspect because officials were not actually classifying the motives of people who were taking their own life, but were classifying their own ideas about the motives of suicides. He recognized that the officials' particularized operational definitions shaped their categorizations, causing their classifications of motive to not necessarily match the actual motives of the suicide victim. Durkheim, however, did not apply this same critique to the categorizations of *types of death,* that is, whether the death was a suicide, accident, homicide, or was due to "natural" means. Perhaps this was because Durkheim needed suicide motives to be *problematic* in order that they might be explained within his theoretical structure, while he needed to keep the suicide statistics *intact* in order to have an objective base for his theoretical structure. Durkheim has also been accused of keeping the official suicide statistics intact only when they fitted his theory and explaining them away when they did not so fit.[8]

It is certainly the case that the sociologist cannot naively assume that the definitions of suicide with which he is operating are the same as those being used by officials who categorize deaths. Nor does it seem adequate to dispense with the problem by merely mentioning it and then continuing to accept the official statistics *as though* they did, in fact, have this match. It is refreshing to note that Verkko,[39] the director of the National Bureau of Statistics in Finland, has written on the problem of utilizing different meanings of suicide, especially the problem of incorporating premeditated and nonpremeditated acts into the same category. How, we might ask, do statistics vary from one region to another on the basis of just this single aspect of differential categorization? Or even within the same region over time as different officials take office? And yet the usual assumption by sociologists is that the match is *sufficient* to both derive and test hypotheses.

A major problem with Durkheim's use of official suicide statistics and his categorization of suicidal deaths has received previous attention.[2,8,19] While Durkheim defines "altruistic suicide" as one of his major types of suicidal deaths, officials systematically exclude such deaths from their statistics. In Western culture, what Durkheim called "altruistic suicide" is not typically called suicide at all, but rather goes under an entirely different commonsense classification, such as "one who heroically gave up his life that others might live" or some such nonsuicidal category.[21] If for no other reason, this should be enough to make us seriously question our uncritical use of official statistics.

As a further example, we can cite the following case of the father of a 25-year-old man who shot himself. The behavior of this father illustrates how the stigma of classifying a death as suicide can be a driving force in interpersonal behavior:

(The father) first blamed the police department for purposely hiding information and for filing a false police report. He attributed as motive for such action that "half the police department laid the girl (his son) was going with, and the department had to protect itself." He accused his son's girlfriend of knowing more than she admitted, intimating a plot between her and her husband for insurance money. He attempted to have an inquest held to determine the cause of his son's death, but was refused the inquest when the coroner stated that he was satisfied with the police report. He then accused the coroner of having ulterior motives in his decision. Finally, he attempted to have the F.B.I. brought in to investigate the case, but he failed in this also when the F.B.I. informed him that they would have to have a basis for investigating the entire police department if they were to enter any such case[20] [pp. 209-210].

The point of this example is that suicide is still a terrible stigma in our society; thus, there is basis for strong motives to make certain that a death is classified in a particular way, in this case, to push the death into some category other than suicide.

If the social meaning of suicide is so strong that it can motivate or even compel an interested party to take the drastic steps described in the previous case, might this not be a common factor to consider in suicides in our culture? And might it not have a systematic effect on the categorizing of suicide? Sociologists should especially make problematic the question of how the social meaning of suicide can lead to systematic bias in the official statistics on which they so heavily rely. Although the father in this case was unsuccessful in his attempts at influencing the categorization of death, we must note that he was a common working man, a millwright with an approximate income of $11,000. This leads us to relevant sociological questions concerning the possible effects of social class differentials in power in determining suicide statistics. How, for example, might the above case been handled differently by the officials if the suicide's father had been from the upper class? At the minimum, there most certainly would have been a thorough investigation, with the additional possibility that the coroner would have been less likely to categorize the death as a suicide in the first place.

Not only might differential social class pressure and influence affect suicide statistics, but how might collusion fit into the picture? How might the meaning of death by suicide be built into the official statistics of different regions of the country? How might a dominant religion in a particular area affect its official suicide statistics? When Henslin applied for a post-doctoral fellowship at Harvard to study the adjustment of families of suicides, it was pointed out to him that the official statistics of suicide in the Boston area were probably extremely inaccurate. With Boston's high proportion of Roman Catholics and its Catholic-dominated politics (coroners are usually political officials), it is likely that the official statistics are systematically biased against Roman Catholics showing up with a high rate, leading to concomitant relative disproportions in the official Protestant suicide rate.

With Roman Catholics, this biasing process begins with the family's desire to remove stigma from the deceased and themselves, with the desire for a "blessed" death that will not generate any questions about where the deceased can be buried. At least we don't drive a wooden stake through the hearts of suicide victims and then confiscate their property, as was once done in England, but there are still questions in some instances about where individuals of the Roman Catholic faith who commit suicide may be buried. It is also necessary to consider the family doctor, who might also be a Roman Catholic who shares the stigmatizing meaning of suicide. Out of his concern for the well-being of the survivors, he has a vested interest in declaring the death something other than a suicide. Who knows but that the overdose might not actually have been accidental? And the threat of the night before, merely jest?

This illustrates only a single dimension of shared meanings that probably tends to systematically bias official suicide statistics. Yet, fascinatingly enough, most sociologists blithely assume that such factors either do not exist, or that if they do, they are not significant. This example deals with only the question of the vested interest of the family's *religion* and the categorization of suicide. When we add such variables as social class, with concomitant differences in power to influence officials, the situation quickly becomes even more complicated. And when we try to compare cross-cultural statistics, the situation becomes almost impossible. If we cannot even assume unidimensionality of meaning in the categorization of death among American coroners, how can we attempt to make such an assumption regarding officials in other cultures, who probably approach their task with contrasting sets of definitions? It certainly appears more logical to assume that operational definitions are multidimensional. Yet, sociologists regularly make cross-cultural comparisons of official suicide rates, culled from United Nations published data, and expect that these will demonstrate some aspect of some pet sociological theory. And, indeed they do illustrate theory, but not sociological theory concerning suicide. Rather, their use clearly reflects sociological thinking, or nonthinking, concerning the production of official statistics.

The best current example of a *critical* approach to suicide statistics is in the operation of the Los Angeles Suicide Prevention Center. Here the staff does not routinely and unquestioningly accept the classification of deaths by coroners. Their experience has taught them that such an approach is naive at best and can be exceedingly misleading. The Los Angeles Coroner's Office has hired behavioral scientists to serve as deputy coroners. Each equivocal death is investigated by a team of researchers who jointly discuss in a seminar the evidence they have uncovered and the results of the interviews that they have held with significant others.[26, 31, 41] On the basis of such evidence and conferences, decisions as to the mode of death are made. Among other things, these *psychological autopsies,* as they are called, could certainly serve as examples for the development of *sociological autopsies.* Additionally, they might lead to the development of sound evidence from which productive theories could be derived. At a minimum, the practices of the Los Angeles Suicide Prevention Center give empirical support to the position that official suicide statistics should not be unquestioningly accepted as fact, and that they are indeed an extremely poor base upon which to generate or test sociological theory.

In criticizing official suicide statistics, one can go too far with the emphasis on meaning. Douglas, for example, comes close to the position that there is really no such thing as suicide. He emphasizes the meaning of the actor who dies to such a degree that at one point,[8] he appears to say that categorizing a corpse as "dead" is an unfair, biased, and ethnocentric attribution if the actor, such as *ronin* of Japan or Asian Buddhists, meant to gain life through his act. If we take the phenomenological position to such an extreme that we must always accept the actor's definition of his act as the only valid definition, then those who take their own lives are not to be considered suicides if they believe their action will lead to greater life. If the extreme phenomenological position is valid, then an actor who says that he isn't committing suicide, yet dies by his own hand, has not in fact committed suicide. Such a point of view appears to us to be taking the phenomenological position to ludicrous extremes. Although intentions differ, death is an objective fact, and corpses can be counted. In determining whether a death is a suicide or not, we must surely consider the definitions and intentions of the deceased, but in our conceptualizations of suicide we also have some objective things to deal with. On the other hand, we think that the "that's-all-we-have" argument concerning official statistics is extremely inadequate and that sociologists should critically examine them in order to determine how the deaths about which they theorize are categorized.[5]

Suicide Rates

As an example of the unquestioning use of official suicide statistics by sociologists, let us look at a study by Labovitz.[24] He follows the usual procedure of first stating that suicide rates are unreliable, but then he tests his hypotheses as though an angel from heaven had delivered the data in sealed and uncontaminated containers. Although Labovitz states that he knows suicide statistics are unreliable, he still insists on attempting to explain official suicide statistics on the basis of some underlying suicide rate that they supposedly illustrate, and not on the basis of the problematic nature of the statistics themselves.

As Labovitz examines century old suicide statistics (See Table 1.), he comes across some that are unexpected. However, instead of even suggesting

TABLE 1 — Suicide Rates for Selected Countries, Nineteenth Century

Country	Suicide Rate	Period	Suicide Rate	Period	Suicide Rate	Period
Saxony	39	1878-82	20	1847-51		
Denmark	25	1881-85	26	1845-56	22	1835-44
Prussia	20	1881-85	11	1849-52		
France	19	1881-84	10	1849-54	8	1935-43
Sweden	10	1881-85	7	1840-50	6	1825-40
Belgium	8	1871-80	6	1841-50		
Norway	7	1881-85	11	1846-55		

Adapted from Karen Dreyer, "Comparative Suicide Statistics," *Danish Medical Bulletin*, 6: 67, 1959 and as contained in Labovitz[24] p. 62.

that such unexpected suicide rates might be artifacts of the suicide statistics gathering process, he accepts them as representing realities to be explained. Using statistics that cover only a 31 year period in one country (Sweden) and even shorter temporal periods in other countries (for example, 1847 to 1851 and 1878 to 1882—a mere ten years—in the case of Saxony), Labovitz draws the somewhat amazing conclusion that "the statistics suggest a substantial increase in the suicide rate through the century."[24] Not only do these statistics fail to cover the whole century in the first place, but when three out of seven countries do not go in the predicted direction, these are taken as "exceptions to be explained." Not once is it suggested that these statistics from the 19th century are probably meaningless as far as representing any so-called "true" suicide rate, that instead of representing actual rates these figures might represent the methods used to gather statistics on suicide.

By this example we do not mean to merely cite the misuse of statistics, but to also indicate that suicide statistics themselves are suspect. As a further example, look at Table 2 in which more recent statistics are utilized.

These statistics are again accepted as representing some so-called true suicide rate, some reality to be explained. It is, however, quite possible that this table of suicide rates contains meaning not related to suicide rates at all. For example, to this data we can apply the following simple theorems and hypothesis:

Theorem One: "The more industrialized or literate a country, the more emphasis it places on bookkeeping procedures."
Theorem Two: "Official suicide statistics represent the degree of emphasis on bookkeeping procedures."
Theorem Three: "Less industrialized and/or less literate areas of the world demonstrate lower official suicide statistics."
Hypothesis: "Central and South America will exhibit a low rate of suicide, as measured by their official suicide statistics."

We made this set of theorems and this hypothesis prior to an examination of Table 2, thus following "good scientific procedure." In examining this table, we see that the countries representative of Central and South America (Chile, Colombia, Costa Rica, Dominican Republic, Guatemala, Panama, and Peru) have a mean suicide rate of 2.44 for 1952 and 3.88 for 1962, while the mean suicide rate for the other countries represented in the table is 10.7 for 1952 and 11.6 for 1962. These differences are significant at the .01 level for *both* years using a test for means.

Although our hypothesis is substantiated statistically, we do not contend that it has been demonstrated. We mean to make the point, rather, that it can frequently be more profitable to develop hypotheses concerning the gathering of official suicide statistics than to develop hypotheses concerning what these statistics supposedly represent about some actual suicide rate.

TABLE 2 — Suicide Rates for 38 Countries, Circa 1952 and 1962

Country	Circa 1952	Circa 1962
Australia	10.6	15.7
Austria	23.4	21.7
Belgium	13.1	13.6
Bulgaria	7.4	8.4
Canada	7.3	7.6
Ceylon	6.9	9.7
Chile	4.3	6.6
China (Taiwan)	1.0	1.8
Colombia	1.6	5.0
Costa Rica	2.6	3.7
Denmark	22.9	19.0
Dominican Republic	3.3	1.0
England and Wales	9.9	12.2
Finland	17.6	19.2
France	15.5	15.5
Germany, West	17.7	19.3
Guatemala	1.8	3.1
Hungary	17.8	26.8
Iceland	11.5	7.6
Ireland	2.2	2.5
Italy	6.3	5.5
Japan	18.5	15.9
Luxembourg	8.9	9.3
Mexico	0.9	1.8
Netherlands	6.3	6.2
New Zealand	10.1	9.6
Norway	6.9	7.9
Panama	2.9	6.4
Peru	0.6	1.4
Poland	5.4	9.3
Portugal	9.2	9.6
Puerto Rico	12.4	7.4
Scotland	5.5	8.6
Spain	5.9	5.2
Sweden	16.7	18.5
Switzerland	21.5	18.5
Union of South Africa		
Asiatic	13.0	9.3
Coloured	1.6	3.8
White	9.3	17.1
United States	10.0	11.0

Source: *Demographic Yearbook,* 1964, New York: United Nations, 1965, Table 22 as contained in Labovitz[24] p. 61.

It might be interesting if various other hypotheses were applied to such official rates, such as, for example: Countries that are predominantly Roman Catholic will demonstrate lower suicide rates than non-Roman Catholic countries, basing this hypothesis *not* on the Durkheimian notion that Roman Catholics commit suicide less frequently because of some so-called "solidarity" within their religion, but, rather, on the notion that due to their religion, Roman Catholics have a greater vested interest in concealing suicide (as in the previous Boston example), and their official suicide statistics represent this concealment. Perhaps we can even talk about such things as *concealment rates* and it might even be possible that we can establish a hypothesis on the need for particular social groups to conceal suicide rates. This might be a rather interesting concept to apply to official suicide statistics. In any event, it is unlikely to be worthwhile to play the "statistics game" in any way whatsoever because of the current state of these official statistics. Yet, some sociologists insist that such criticisms are merely carping and that we should continue our uncritical use of official suicide rates.[16]

A profitable direction for sociologists to take as they study suicide would be to concentrate on the rate-making process itself. A phenomenological approach to the decision making process of coroners, it seems to us, would prove invaluable in determining actual rates of suicide. By investigating the factors that a coroner uses to make his decisions, and comparing these from coroner to coroner, we may be able to better determine such things as the relationship between the social class of the decedent and the coroner's decision regarding cause of death, the effects of a family's religion on the coroner's decision, or even the effects of the coroner's own religion on his decision. Additionally, the organizational factors that may play a role in the decision making process could and should be investigated. Especially, how do various differential guidelines provided by his county or state or differential requisite qualifications for holding the position of coroner, lead to differential defining in similar situations? What everyday presuppositions and expectations does a coroner follow in problematic situations, such rules based not only on his training but also on his own group memberships—sexual, social class, religious, racial, age, and even geographical? The phenomenological study of such rate-making processes is not limited to suicide, of course, but is crucial to the understanding of many forms of deviance, such as crime, delinquency, and mental illness.[5]

The statement that sociologists should "get into the 'real world' " has become somewhat hackneyed, but it appears to us that this is the direction that sociologists who study suicide must take. It is time for us to move away from unreliable official indicators of suicide rates and to actually begin the study of suicide, that is if we hope to progress somewhat more in the next hundred years than we have in the past hundred.

Unicausality and Unidimensionality of Suicide

Sociologists from Durkheim to the present have sought a single common denominator to explain suicide rates. Recently a sociologist has even attempted to reconceptualize Durkheim's theory of suicide into a unicausal theory.[22] Johnson eliminates Durkheim's concepts of egoism and fatalism as nonessential, and he also states that the concepts of egoism and anomie are indistinguishable. He then says that Durkheim's theory can be succinctly restated as: "The more integrated (regulated) a society, group or social condition is, the lower its suicide rate." Others have taken social disorganization as the unicausal factor behind suicide rates, for example, Benedict,[1] Cavan,[4] Dublin and Bunzel,[9] Elliot and Merrill,[12] Faris,[3] Mowrer,[29] and Schmid.[36, 37] The problem common to those who have looked for a unicausal theory to explain suicide is that they have had extreme difficulty in operationalizing whatever causal variable they have chosen. There is, for example, extreme disagreement on the operational meaning of social disorganization. Where Durkheim failed to operationalize his concepts, sociologists following his wake have usually tried to do so, but they have unfortunately failed to establish adequate definitions.

These theorists usually make explicit the view that suicide is a negative act. Implicit in their arguments and theories is that suicide, accordingly, must be caused by a prior negative event. It is possible that this basic assumption is not valid; if we do not start with such a guiding assumption, the possibility of a different type of suicide emerges. For example, perhaps success rather than failure is the basic cause of some types of suicide. While it might be difficult for us to conceptualize this, we should not proceed on the unexamined assumption that it is not true.

It is possible that a variety of explanations of suicide must be proposed, although it has been argued[8] that a multicausal explanation will blanket diverse instances of suicide. Whatever the case, there is currently no single concept[24, 27] present in sociology that can account for the variation in suicide rates as they are measured by official statistics. Labovitz[24] suggests that we "must postulate a common denominator or factor that distinguishes all populations with high rates. This factor, if one exists, appears unrelated to conventional sociological concepts or commonly recognized social distinctions."

It is possible, however, that the reason that we do not presently have a unidimensional sociological concept to explain suicide is not due to the lack of imagination or conceptualizing by sociologists who have studied suicide, but due to the fact that suicide itself is not an unidimensional phenomenon. It is quite probable that the category suicide, although appearing to be the same thing in all cases envelops different phenomena under a single umbrella. Perhaps the meaning of the actor must be taken into account if we are to adequately explain or understand suicide. For example, suicide might be due to hostility, aggression, frustration, revenge, to the desire to hurt another person or even to prevent hurt to other persons. Suicide may also be due to "suicide gestures" that have gone wrong; that is, to suicide attempts which were not meant to be completed but which became "accidentally successful." For example, a housewife may be extremely disgusted and upset with her life situation and deteriorating relationship with her husband. In an attempt to win sympathy from him and to bring about a change in her life situation, she takes pills she knows take a certain amount of time to take effect. She takes them a few minutes before her husband is expected home, knowing that for the past twenty years he has come home at the same time every day. Yet, on this particular day, he is unexpectedly detained by overtime at the factory, or by traffic.

Once one identifies different types of suicide, the possibility is opened that these types have entirely *different causes*. Instead of assuming unidimensionality, perhaps sociologists should begin with the working assumption that suicide is multidimensional. We then face the interesting possibility that there might not only be different causes but also different rates for different types of suicide.

In their attempt to find a unicausal theory of suicide, and in their use of suicide statistics, sociologists have sometimes developed theories that are at least partially tautological. For example, Gibbs and Porterfield[18] have developed a theory of the relationship between experiencing crises and committing suicide.[8] They incorporate the idea of crisis into their theory of status change: individuals who experience mobility in the social structure, either up or down, experience changes in supportive social relations such that when they experience a crisis, their probability of committing suicide is increased compared with persons who have not experienced the status change and are confronted by a crisis. When actual cases of suicide are examined, strong support is given to this theory. But what is overlooked in this reasoning is that part of the operational definition used by officials in deciding whether a particular death is suicide, accident, homicide, or natural is whether the deceased had experienced a crisis shortly before his death. If they find that he did, the chances increase that his death will be labeled suicide; if a crisis cannot be located, the chance that his death will be classified into one of the other categories increases. Thus, when faced by a problematic death, a coroner looks for crises, and if he finds one, he is more likely to assume that the death was by suicide than he would have been otherwise. This leads to the common newspaper accounts of problematic deaths that are labeled as suicides: for example, "Mr. Jones had been despondent in recent weeks because of the loss of his (wife, mother, grandmother, sister, daughter, son, father, uncle, job, or parakeet)." It is not surprising, then, that the sociologist will find that which the coroner tries to make certain is present.

It is rare for a sociologist to make a direct statement to explain what differentiates the person who does commit suicide from the one who does not. The only such statement that we have come across is made by Gibbs.[14] He says, "all suicide victims have experienced a set of disrupted social relationships not found in the history of nonvictims." Gibbs surely does not mean to say that *all* suicide victims have experienced *more* "disrupted social relationships," for we could then get some measurement of the number of such disruptions, and his theory would be easily falsifiable. He must therefore be referring to the *quality* of such "social disruptions" which takes us back to our unresolved problem of operationalization.

Gibbs does, in fact, specify the need for knowing the *amount* and *type,* as well as the *timing* and *anticipating* of disruptions. However, as he says, as long as such a statement is not operationalized and tested, it remains just what it appears to be, merely an assertion, and no theory at all. Gibbs is making a good attempt to state that there *is* something that differentiates the suicide victim from the non-suicide victim, but with our present state of measurement in sociology, much less our current state of conceptualization, such an attempt is indeed abortive.

Although Gibbs is fully aware that a theory must be operationalized and testable in order to be confirmed or disconfirmed, he points to a problem that has plagued sociologists in their study of suicide: an adequate theory must meet the major criterion of being refutable or falsifiable.[32] Durkheim failed to give any clear-cut measures by which his theory could be confirmed or disconfirmed and thus made his theory irrefutable. The same criticism can be laid at the door of sociologists who have written on suicide in recent years. Gibbs and Martin[17] propose a status-integration theory of suicide in which they (1) take stability and durability of social relationships as a measure of social integration, (2) take amount of role conflict as a measure of the durability and stability of social relationships, and (3) take status as a measure of role. Unfortunately, they do not define status,[8] leaving their theory untestable and, accordingly, of very little value.

Overview of Sociological Theories of Suicide

Various sociological theories concerning suicide have been put forth. These can be summarized as follows[28] [pp. 8-91]:

Theorist	Theory
Halbwachs	The suicide rate varies directly with the degree of social isolation.
Halbwachs	The suicide rate varies directly with the degree of urbanization.
Henry and Short; Maris	The suicide rate varies inversely with the degree of external restraint placed on behavior.
Henry and Short	The suicide rate varies directly with status.
Gibbs and Martin	The suicide rate varies inversely with the degree of status integration.
Durkheim; Gibbs and Martin	The suicide rate varies inversely with stability and durability of social relationships.
Durkheim; Johnson	The suicide rate varies inversely with the degree of integration.
Durkheim; Johnson	The suicide rate varies directly with the degree of anomie.

176

Morselli	The suicide rate varies directly with the degree of civilization.
Schmid	The suicide rate varies directly with the degree of social disorganization.
Porterfield	The suicide rate varies directly with the degree of secularization.
Dublin and Bunzel	The suicide rate varies inversely with the degree of societal condemnation of suicide.

Common to these theories is that they all fail to clearly state the assumed underlying relations between the dependent and independent variables. Additionally, these theories come under the criticisms we have just discussed. They are not falsifiable since adequate procedures are typically not specified for measuring the independent variable. In order to adequately test a theory, the theory must generate at least one empirical proposition which is logically possible to be refuted.[32] If it is impossible to refute (falsify) a theory, its empirical value cannot be tested.

Some of these theories also rest on very shaky assumptions, such as Henry and Short's assumption that "the strength of social relational systems is greater among rural residents than urban residents, among married persons than among unmarried, and among persons living in outlying areas of large cities than among residents of centrally located areas." As Martin[28] points out, these judgments are primarily based on *folklore* about the social relations of these populations. Additionally, these theorists of suicide causation are frequently forced to shift their position in order to account for discrepancies between the official suicide rates and their hypotheses. For example, Henry and Short[28] appear to reverse their position on "status" and "strength of a relational system" in accounting for the suicide rate of the aged and the married.

The tremendous and fascinating overlap and lack of originality of these theories should be apparent when we summarize them. They state that the rate of suicide varies *directly* with the degree of:

Civilization
Urbanization
Status
Social disorganization
Secularization
Social isolation
Anomie
and *inversely* with:
External restraint
Societal integration
Status integration
Stability and durability of social relationships, and
Social condemnation of suicide [p. 84].

Such theories might turn out to be real "work horses," for (sometimes by merely changing "directly" to read "inversely" and vice versa), they appear to be just as easily applied in the explanation of such disparate and sometimes troubling aspects of modern social life as divorce, burglary, rape, death by fire, public intoxication, the incidence of skid row alcoholism, personal property values and their fluctuations over time as measured by "official fluctuation rates," literacy rates, the number of papers presented at sociological conventions, the incidence of fingernail biting, the number of books published on marine life, amount of income, amount of gross national product, the likelihood of campus disruptions, riots, or even participation in national revolution. But, again, just "what" is "explained" by such theories?

It is possible to multiply such unicausal theories *ad infinitum*. For example, one could hypothesize that the following are "causes" of the suicide rate: mental instability; weakness of mind; irresolution or vacillation in meeting life's problems; fatalism; independence; individualism; relations with parents, children, spouse, or lovers; happiness; happy-go-luckiness; and moodiness. In fact, these are probably just as good concepts and theories as the ones we currently have, since we are also unable to satisfactorily operationalize and test them.

SOCIAL MEANINGS OF SUICIDE

To discover the basis for imputed consistencies which might underlie suicide rates of social groups, for example, occupational groups, we cannot look only at external life factors for the explanation. Different people may face the same external life situation, such as divorce or loss of wealth, and some will commit suicide, while the vast majority will not. If we attribute cause to such factors, we can easily fall into the ecological fallacy. We must look beyond the external, so-called "objective" life situation of individuals and examine the symbolic system within which objective situations are mediated. In other words, we must look at the system within which the individual attributes meaning to events and then decides on or rejects suicide.

Douglas[8] interprets Durkheim as taking social meanings as the fundamental cause of suicide, saying that Durkheim argues that social meanings underly social behavior and as such are the ultimate causes of suicide. Durkheim looks on men interacting together as producing social meanings which remain stable within individuals and cause their actions. This gives rise to the fact that some groups, having differing pools of meanings, have different suicide rates.

Durkheim says that society needs a balance in its members among submissive, aloof, and rebellious organizations. An imbalance in the equilibrium of these three orientations produces the proportion of individuals who tend toward suicide, resulting in a group's particular suicide rate. This disequilibrium stems from a variety of experiences in human associations, for example, economic failure occurs with different frequencies and intensities in certain social groups.

Because of collective nature of experiences, the same external events may have dissimilar meaning for different persons. Collectively shared meaning mediates experiences and disposes people toward or away from suicide. As has been argued, Durkheim only paid lip service to a positivistic approach and made his data fit his ideas where necessary; he repeats this error when he attempts to determine the various meanings that social experiences have for different groups. Thus, when his theory would indicate that suicide increases as education increases, he then comes across a fact that doesn't fit (for example, Jews have both high education and low suicide), he posits a different meaning regarding education for the Jew than for the Protestant. He does not, however, provide any test for the accuracy of the meaning he posits; he actually substitutes *his* ideas of what things mean for the meanings the things have for the persons in the particular groups. In other words, to test his theory, Durkheim used his common-sense understandings based on his everyday experiences.[8]

The most complete analysis of the role of "meanings" in the process of suicide has been made by Douglas[8] who, in our opinion, makes an excellent case for the need of understanding the meaning of the actor in order to understand the phenomena of suicide. A more recent attempt to do this is made by Henslin.[21] By utilizing emphases in the ethnomethodological and ethnoscientific approaches to the study of human behavior, Henslin indicates that cultural bases of perception must be examined if suicide is to be understood. The effects of cultural categories in determining meanings of death, particularly that of suicide, must be thoroughly examined by suicide researchers. Through culturally-provided categories of death, as well as through subcultural experiences, meaning is given to suicide. Meanings in general stem from fitting objects, events, and interactions into such culturally-provided categories. Placing events into categories yields explanations, orientations, and interpretations, since "explanatory orientations" are not contained in the event itself. Although these papers by Henslin deal primarily with families of those who have had a member commit suicide, the principles that he utilizes can also be applied to persons who face various problems in living, to those who contemplate suicide, and to persons who have attempted suicide. These papers are exploratory, and being only suggestive, much further research needs to be done on suicide phenomena in order to test the fruitfulness of this suggested direction.

Similiar to the use of official suicide statistics, however, validity problems arise when one examines the meaning-content of social phenomena. As Faris[13] indicates:

The farther the investigator pursues contextual meanings in specific unique persons and events, the greater the perils of subjectivity, the more difficulties of reliability and validity, and the more restricted the possible generalizations that can be made. If two sensitive investigators of the same case produce contrasting interpretations, how do we know which is right, or if either is? [p. 643].

Although this danger is present, it appears to us that one cannot adequately understand suicide apart from understanding meanings—meanings for the individual who commits suicide, meanings for the coroner or other officials who decide whether a death is a "suicide," as well as meanings for the survivors. In order to do this, we need much greater research on cultural, subcultural, and personalistic or individuated influences on the meaning phenomena associated with death and suicide.

It appears to us that the vast majority of sociologists who have theorized and otherwise written on suicide *have not actually studied suicide*. They have, instead, studied suicide statistics. It is our position that it would be much more fruitful to research the process of suicide. To understand the suicide process we must understand the ways in which biographical events are mediated through a symbolic system. We must research the ways in which people interpret biographical events and develop meaning systems such that some individuals, when confronted with given situations remove themselves by means of suicide, while others so confronted react differently.

Sociologists must develop methods to tap this suicide process, methods to get at the meanings of events, including that of suicide, for both the victim and his significant others. For instance, one might focus on how the individual ordinarily responded to significant losses in his life to see if patterns of typical response are unique among those who do commit suicide. We must ask why suicide is *not* the alternative chosen by most people when they confront divorce, the death of a significant other, financial disaster, and status change, as well as asking the more obvious question of why people choose suicide.

It is obvious that characteristics common to a group do not lead to suicide, for example, social characteristics such as ruptured primary relations and financial reversals. If they did, we could anticipate that all those experiencing the imputed causal characteristics would commit suicide. Not even the most committed unicausal theorist would make such a claim, however. Thus, suicide is perhaps due to characteristics of which we now know very little. Perhaps our measuring instruments are so crude that these characteristics do not show up; it would appear to now be our task to attempt to develop more sensitive instruments.

Or perhaps a response of suicide is due to the individualized meanings assigned by the person who is experiencing them. Again, it is the sociologist's task, if he desires to understand suicide and break out of his statistical bind, to study the symbolic processes associated with suicide.

Studies of successful suicides are usually characterized by retrospective

180

material supplied by *third persons,* subject to all the pitfalls of such data collection. The researcher is prevented from getting at the meaning of suicide to the person who committed it, except through recollection by these third persons. In order to get around this, we suggest that sociologists begin a concentrated study of those who attempt suicide, using a sample of nonattemptors, matched on variables of life problems confronted as well as on background characteristics. The suicide rate is much higher among those who have once attempted suicide compared with those who have never attempted suicide, with "the incidence of completed suicide among suicide attemptors ranging from .03 to 22 per cent, depending to some extent of the length of the follow up."[7] Thus, by tapping a group highly prone to suicide, we would be including persons who will actually end up dying by means of suicide. In this way, we would gather in-depth data on persons who commit suicide. We could then compare these findings with those gathered from those who attempted but who did not commit suicide, as well as with the nonattemptors. In this way, we would hopefully be able to understand the suicide process.

It is recognized, of course, that such a study of suicide contains many problems. The population of those who attempt suicide is, first of all, not representative of all suicides. Concealment, for example, is a vital aspect of those who attempt suicide: the stigma associated with attempted suicide is an important factor motivating actors to conceal such attempts. Accordingly, selecting a representative population of attemptors becomes most difficult since many of them are unknown.

There is also the ethical problem of studying a population of persons of whom as many as 20 per cent may eventually commit suicide. One does not know whether depth interviews would be therapeutic or whether they might actually precipitate suicide. It also appears that it would be most difficult for a researcher not to drift into the role of therapist when he is dealing with persons confronting severe problems; in such an event, the researcher might actually become the major intervening variable in his research design. Certainly such an approach is extremely complex in many ways, and being longitudinal, it would be very expensive in energy, time, and interest. But such designs appear necessary if sociologists are going to move away from suicide rates and actually begin the study of suicide. This approach, in spite of its problems, would allow us to analyze the suicide process itself, from which we would be able to derive hypotheses that could then be tested on the suicide population.

CONCLUSION

After approximately 75 years of sociological research into suicide, what can sociologists actually say about it? Rushing[35] has given an overview of various theoretical approaches in suicide research, and examined numerous correlates of suicide. He concludes with the following evaluation of what we currently know about it:

Extensive research findings suggest that suicide is associated with physical illness, mental illness, alcoholism, homicide, and economic failure, all of which tend to result in disruptions in social relations. Suicide is also related to the communication of intent. The most general conclusion is, then, that interpersonal elements, particularly disruptive social relations, are crucial etiological factors in suicide [p. 121].

And *that* is just about where the field of sociology is today. Disruptive interpersonal elements lead to suicide. Not much to show for 75 years of research.

We have, unfortunately, wasted valuable years and effort utilizing statistics that are worth very little. Yet many sociologists continue this pattern today, publishing small studies that purport to demonstrate some aspect or other about suicide. Perhaps this is because they have a readily available journal market, and it helps to satisfy the "publish or perish" dictum under which university employed sociologists labor. But these studies are based on suicide statistics that were gathered with a different operational definition than the researcher has, and, in spite of their sophisticated-looking statistical tests, drawings, and multicelled tables,[22] they go very little beyond Durkheim's *Suicide* of over 70 years ago. It is entirely possible that Durkheim unwittingly did a great disservice to the advancement of sociology by writing *Suicide* since it has blinded sociologists for about three generations. The fault, of course, lies not with Durkheim but with his unimaginative followers who could not break away from the unfruitful path that he pioneered. Just as it is sometimes difficult for an adolescent to cut maternal apronstrings, so it is sometimes difficult for those following a pioneer in academia to objectively appraise the worth of his contribution, since they feel that they owe much to him and they tend to identify so strongly with what he left behind. But although difficult, it is frequently necessary—if the discipline is to progress. And progress it must, or remain forever encapsulated in the incrustation of the thought-framework of its founders.

REFERENCES

1. BENEDICT, R.: *Patterns of Culture.* Boston: Houghton Mifflin, 1934.
2. BENOIT-SMULLYAN, E.: "The Sociologism of Emile Durkheim and His School," in Harry E. Barnes (ed.): *An Introduction to the History of Sociology.* Chicago: University of Chicago Press, 1948, Pp. 205-243.
3. BOISMONT, B., DE: *Du Suicide et de la Folie Suicide.* Paris: Bailliere, 1856.
4. CAVAN, R. S.: *Suicide.* Chicago: University of Chicago Press, 1928.
5. CHAPPELL, D., GEIS, G., SCHAEFER, S., AND SIEGEL, L.: "Forcible Rape: A Comparative Study of Offenses Known to the Police in Boston and Los Angeles," in James M. Henslin (ed.): *The Sociology of Sex: A Book of Original Studies.* New York: Appleton-Century-Crofts, 1971, pp. 169-190.
6. DE GURREY, *Statisque Morale de la France,* in Jack Douglas (ed.). *The Meanings in Suicide.* Princeton, New Jersey: Princeton University Press, 1967, p. 171.

7. DORPAT, T. L., AND JOHNSON, M.: "The Relationship Between Attempted and Committed Suicide." *Comprehensive Psychiatry* 8: as cited in Rushing 1968:99, 1967.

8. DOUGLAS, J. D.: *The Social Meanings of Suicide.* Princeton, New Jersey: Princeton University Press, 1967.

9. DUBLIN, L. I., AND BUNZEL, B.: *To Be or Not To Be.* New York: Harrison, Smith, and Robert Hass, 1933.

10. DURKHEIM, E.: *The Division of Labor in Society.* Translated and with an introduction by George Simpson. New York: The Macmillan Company. (First published in 1893.), 1933.

11. DURKHEIM, E.: *Suicide: A Study in Sociology.* Translated by John A. Spaulding and George Simpson. Edited and with an introduction by George Simpson. New York: The Free Press of Glencoe, Inc. (First published in 1897.), 1951.

12. ELLIOTT, M. L., AND MERRILL, F. E.: *Social Disorganization.* New York: Harper and Row, 1941.

13. FARIS, R. E.: *Social Disorganization.* New York: The Ronald Press Company, 1968.

14. GIBBS, J. P.: (Ed.) *Suicide.* New York: Harper and Row, 1968.

15. GIBBS, J. P.: "Suicide," in Robert K. Merton and Robert A. Nisbet (eds.): *Contemporary Social Problems: An Introduction to the Sociology of Deviant Behavior and Social Disorganization.* New York: Harcourt, Brace, and World, Inc. 1961, Pp. 222-261.

16. GIBBS, J. P.: Book review of *The Social Meanings of Suicide* by Jack D. Douglas. *The American Journal of Sociology,* 74: 201-204, 1968.

17. GIBBS, J. P., AND MARTIN, W. T.: "A Theory of Status Integration and Its Relationship to Suicide." *American Sociological Review* 23: 140-147, 1958.

18. GIBBS, J. P., AND PORTERFIELD, A. L.: "Occupational Prestige and Social Mobility of Suicides in New Zealand." *American Journal of Sociology* 46: 147-152, 1960.

19. HALBWACHS, M.: *Les Cause du Suicide.* Paris: Felix Alcan, 1930.

20. HENSLIN, J. M.: "Guilt and Guilt Neutralization: Response and Adjustment to Suicide," in Jack D. Douglas (ed.): *Deviance and Respectability: The Social Construction of Moral Meanings.* New York: Basic Books, Inc. 1970, Pp. 192-228.

21. HENSLIN, J. M.: "The Construction of Social Meanings Following a Suicide," in Jack D. Douglas (ed.): *Existential Sociology.* New York: Appleton-Century-Crofts. 1972.

22. JOHNSON, B. D.: "Durkheim's One Cause of Suicide." *American Sociological Review 30:* 875-886, 1965.

23. KINSEY, B. A.: Book review of *Social Forces in Urban Suicide* by Maris. *American Sociological Review* 35: 409, 1970.

24. LABOVITZ, S.: "Variation in Suicide Rates," in Jack P. Gibbs (ed.): *Suicide.* New York: Harper and Row, 1968, Pp. 57-73.

25. LEGOYT, A.: *Suicide Acien et Moderne.* Paris: Drouin, 1881.

26. LITMAN, R. E., CURPHEY, T., SHNEIDMAN, E. S., FARBEROW, N. L., AND TABACHNICK, N.: "Investigations of Equivocal Suicides." 184:924-929, 1963.

27. MARIS, R. W.: *Social Forces in Urban Suicide.* Homewood, Illinois: The Dorsey Press, 1969.

28. MARTIN, W. T.: "Theories of Variation in the Suicide Rates" in Jack P. Gibbs (ed.): *Suicide.* New York: Harper and Row, 1968, Pp. 74-96.

29. MOWRER, E.: *Disorganization: Personal and Social.* Philadelphia: Lippincott, 1942.

29. NISBET, R. A.: *Emile Durkheim.* Englewood Cliffs, New Jersey: Prentice-Hall, Inc. 1965.

31. PECK, M., AND SCHRUT, A.: "Suicidal Behavior among College Students." *H.S.M.H.A. Health Reports* 86: 149-156, 1971.

32. POPPER, K. R.: *The Logic of Scientific Discovery.* New York: Basic Books, 1959.

33. POWELL, E. H.: "Occupation, Status, and Suicide: Toward a Redefinition of Anomie." *American Sociological Review* 23: 131-139, 1958.

34. ROBINSON, W. S.: "Ecological Correlations and the Behavior of Individuals," *American Sociological Review* 15: 351-357, 1950.

35. RUSHING, W. H.: "Individual Behavior and Suicide," in Jack P. Gibbs (ed.): *Suicide.* New York: Harper and Row, 1968, Pp. 96-121.

36. SCHMID, C. F.: *Suicides in Seattle, 1914 to 1925: An Ecological and Behavioristic Study.* Seattle: University of Washington, 1928.

37. SCHMID, C. F.: "Suicide in Minneapolis, Minnesota: 1928-1932." *The American Journal of Sociology* 39:30-48, 1933.

38. Schmid, C. F.: *Suicide in Seattle, Washington, and Pittsburgh, Pennsylvania: A Comparative Study.* Pittsburgh: University of Pittsburg Bulletin 27: 149-157, 1930.
39. Verkko, V.: *Homicides and Suicides in Finland and Their Dependence on National Character.* Kobehaven: G.E.C. Gads Forlag, 39, (as referred to in Douglas 1967).
40. Zorbaugh, H. W.: *Gold Coast and Slum: A Sociological Study of Chicago's Near North Side.* Chicago, Illinois: The University of Chicago Press, 1929.
41. Curphen, T.: "The Psychological Autopsy: The Role of the Forensic Pathologist in the Multi-Disciplinary Approach to Death." *Bulletin of Suicidology*: 39-45, 1968.

CHAPTER 9

Adjustment to Society: Interrelations Among Anomia, Social Class, and Psychiatric Impairment*

ADINA M. REINHARDT
AND ROBERT M. GRAY

Numerous studies attest to the fact that individuals of lower class standing have higher rates of impaired mental health.[10, 20, 23, 40] This appears to be the case in spite of wide differences among the various studies in regard to the size and nature of their sampling procedures and the particular manner of measuring psychiatric impairment. Fried[10] has commented that even though numerous investigations have been conducted, the field of psychiatric sociology still lacks "an adequate theoretical or empirical appreciation of the complex processes that might meaningfully account for the persistent finding that lower social class groups show the highest rates of psychiatric disorder." Furthermore, there has been virtually no effort to link a relationship between social class factors and psychiatric disorder through intervening social or psychological processes.[10] This emphasizes the need for a comprehensive understanding of the dynamics of the social-psychological processes which may intervene between social class and mental health status. The purpose of this chapter is to present the results of a study which investigated the concept, anomia, as an intervening variable between social class and psychiatric impairment, thus providing clues to the dynamic processes underlying this relationship.

The present study stems from selected findings of a group of interrelated epidemiological studies of psychiatric impairment among "normal" populations. For the purposes of this study, a normal person is defined conceptually as an individual who has never been labelled by a medical doctor, psychiatrist or other official societal functionary as mentally or emotionally ill and in need of psychiatric

*The authors wish to thank Melville R. Klauber Ph.D., University of Utah, College of Medicine, for a number of helpful suggestions regarding the statistical analysis of the data presented in this chapter.

treatment. Operationally, the normal individual is one who scores between 0-3 on the Twenty-Two Item Screening Score of Psychiatric Symptoms Indicating Impairment.[17]

The best known of these investigations is the Midtown Manhattan Study which examined the prevalence of mental disturbance in a sample of 1660 normal nonhospitalized Manhattan residents. Two of the Midtown findings which have implications for the present study were that both socioeconomic status and anomia are related to mental disturbance. Shedding additional light on these findings are the disclosures of other investigators,[7, 11, 13, 22, 23, 31] which collectively reveal that a larger proportion of persons in the lower socioeconomic levels have a tendency to be emotionally unstable.

In an attempt carry these findings one step further, the present chapter has four major aims: (1) to review literature concerned with the epidemiology of psychiatric impairment in normal populations with emphasis upon the relationship between social class and psychiatric impairment; (2) to discuss studies which have examined the relationship between impairment and other measures of individual adjustment to society, such as social participation, self-reports of social satisfaction and happiness; (3) to investigate, in a different geographical setting, the inverse relationship found between various indices of social class and psychiatric impairment in past research; (4) to develop additional insights relative to psychiatric impairment by seeking to determine whether or not anomia maintains a relationship with mental disturbance when various indices of socioeconomic status are held constant. Consistent with previous research, both social class standing and anomia are treated as explanatory variables influencing the self-reports of psychophysiological symptomatology of the respondents. The present inquiry was designed to partially replicate research which has shown a strong inverse association between various indices of social class and mental disturbance and to examine the association, if any, between anomia and psychiatric impairment. In addition to these, the authors have raised the following questions: If there is a relationship between anomia and mental disturbance, will this relationship persist within different levels of socioeconomic status? If so, how does the strength of this relationship vary from one level to another?

MAJOR STUDIES OF PSYCHIATRIC IMPAIRMENT

Epidemiology of Psychiatric Impairment in Normal Populations

The two major surveys of psychiatric epidemiology among normal population groups are the Stirling County Study[14, 21, 23] and the Midtown Manhattan Study. [20,40]

The first of these studies was conducted in Stirling County, Nova Scotia, a rural fishing and farming area in one of the Atlantic provinces of Canada. The research task was two-fold. On the one hand, a social science team had the task of identifying by a series of ten indices certain communities that could be said to be highly integrated and another set of communities that, by the same indices, could be regarded as being in various stages of disintegration. The ten indices were as follows: (1) poverty, (2) cultural confusion, (3) secularization, (4) frequency of broken homes, (5) few and weak associations in the group, (6) few and weak leaders, (7) few patterns of recreation and leisure time activity, (8) high frequency of hostile acts and expressions, (9) high frequency of crime and delinquency, and (10) weak and fragmented network of communication. On the other hand, an epidemiological and psychiatric team had to assess the prevalence of psychiatric disorder. Thus, the issue was to determine whether sociocultural disintegration would bring about conditions which would foster psychiatric disorder.

The psychiatric prevalence data was obtained on a systematic ten per cent sample weighted toward heads of households. Multiple techniques and sources of information were used in the assessment of the psychiatric status of the subjects; questionnaires on personal, social and family characteristics, interviews to determine health, medical and psychiatric symptoms, institutional records of lifetime illness, impressions of local physicians, findings in a psychiatric clinic, observations by interviewers, and evaluative classifications by a group of psychiatrists. Finally, four categories of "caseness" (that is, the probability of being a psychiatric case) were established for classifying the respondents.

Of the nine original hypotheses upon which the investigation was focused, the following four were supported. Social disintegration fosters psychiatric disorder (1) by interfering with the achievement of socially valuable ends by legitimate means; (2) by limitations put on the giving and receiving of love; (3) by interfering with spontaneity; and (4) by interfering with the individual's sense of membership in the moral order. The last of these hypotheses, that social disintegration fosters psychiatric disorder by interfering with the individual's sense of membership in the moral order, is particularly pertinent in the present context in that feelings of anomia are a reflection of an individual's lack of a sense of membership in the moral order.

Furthermore, in summarizing some of the findings of the Stirling County Study, Leighton and her associates[22] noted that:

It is not poverty or limited education or lower class status, per se, that makes the difference to mental health, but rather a whole group of factors that tend to be associated with these and that create a social environment that lacks features that are vitally important to mental health. To improve mental health, economic resources must be mobilized up to a point, education must be provided up to a point, but this will not be enough unless these factors bring with them the other environmental forces which add up to giving the individual *the feeling that he is a worthwhile member of a worthwhile group* [p. 1026]. (Emphasis added).

The second major survey of psychiatric epidemiology considered here was conducted in Midtown Manhattan, a typical "Gold Coast and Slum" area with high population density and a heterogeneous population of which "one-third are immigrants, one-third are in-migrants from other cities and towns in the United States, and one-third were born in New York City."[20] The major purpose of the study was the isolation of social and psychological factors associated with different levels of emotional adjustment and different "risks" of becoming mentally ill.

In the Midtown Study, case-finding was conducted through an institutional search and inquiry of private practitioners for residents of that area, and also through home interviews by means of a structured schedule of a 1.5 per cent probability sample of the population of the area aged 20 to 59 years. This sample comprised 1660 individuals. Respondents were asked over 100 questions concerning their psychiatric symptoms. Langner points out that: "In addition to the broad demographic factors there were about 160 items of sociocultural background whose relationship to mental health was tested with socioeconomic status controlled."[18] Approximately one fifth of the items were related to mental health independently of socioeconomic status and these were combined into eight childhood factors and six adult factors. Finally, all information pertaining to each respondent was reviewed and rated by two psychiatrists, who independently prepared mental health ratings from all the information on each subject.

Based on the final ratings, the investigators reported that less than a fifth (approximately 18 per cent) were well, about a third had mild and another fifth had moderate symptoms, and about one quarter were severely impaired.[40] For the major groupings—well, mild to moderate impairment and severe impairment—it is apparent that close agreement between the Stirling County and Midtown Manhattan Studies exists despite the obvious differences in population characteristics relating to urban-rural distribution, ethnic background, and sociocultural factors. However, in both studies, the investigators believe that their impairment rates underestimate the actual occurrence of positive findings.[22,23,40]

Reviewing briefly, we note that the authors had two basic objectives: to determine the true prevalence of mental disorders in the population, and to assess relations between mental disturbances in individuals and sociocultural conditions in their environments. These two objectives bring the key concepts of stress and strain into focus and relate them dynamically to each other. Stress is conceived as being in the sociocultural environment (those environmental forces impinging on an individual) and strain as being in the individual (the individual's reaction to environmental stressors).

Systematic analysis of relations between stress factors and strain show consistently high mental illness probabilities for persons of low socioeconomic status in comparison with those of middle and high status. Furthermore, the data reveal that strain is directly proportional to stress. Finally, persons in the low socioeconomic group report more stress factors than those in the higher socioeconomic groups.

One possible interpretation of these findings is the hypothesis that "the high status group has a more resilient personality . . . . The superior resilience of the high socioeconomic status group may in part come from positive group identification, which we know was a factor in surviving the stress of the Nazi concentration camps."[18] This interpretation, that a sense of positive group identification provides greater resilience to stress quite clearly appears to parallel Leighton's notion concerning the importance for individual mental health of a sense that one is a "worthwhile member of a worthwhile group."[22]

In summary, both the Stirling County and Midtown Studies contain findings having major implications concerning the psychiatrically impairing effect of an individual's lack of a sense of membership in a stable moral order, or a sense of anomia. Thus, it appeared to the present authors that the above interpretations provided general support for Srole's findings concerning the relationship between anomia and mental disturbance. Utilizing early results of the Midtown data, Srole reported that anomia was found to be a corollary of mental disturbance and that, independently of the mental disturbance factor, anomia was a significant corollary of socioeconomic status.[38] Therefore, it seemed of considerable importance to further investigate the relationships between anomia, socioeconomic status, and psychiatric impairment in order to determine whether an individual's lack of a sense of moral integration into the group (anomia) might not, indeed, be an intervening variable between socioeconomic status and psychiatric impairment. If such were found to be the case, anomia might constitute one factor which partially accounts for mental disturbance regardless of social class membership. Before turning to our research data, however, we focus attention on several of the many studies which have revealed strong inverse relationships between various measures of socioeconomic status and psychiatric disorder.

Studies of Social Class and Psychiatric Impairment

In the majority of studies of both treated and untreated mental disorder, the investigators have found a strong inverse relationship between socioeconomic status and psychiatric problems. Hollingshead and Redlich's study of mental illness in New Haven revealed that the prevalence of all disorder was highest in the lowest class and lowest in the upper stratum.[13]

In Leighton's study of Stirling County, occupational level is taken to be roughly indicative of socioeconomic position. Discussing this relationship, the researchers noted that "whatever the cause, psychiatric difficulties seem to be more frequent at the economically lower reaches of the socioeconomic system."[23] The highest prevalence of actual and potential psychiatric disability was found among the lowest group in the occupational hierarchy. This group was comprised of wage workers in agriculture, fishing and forestry.[23] When educational level was employed as an index of socioeconomic status, the relationship between class factors and psychiatric disability was maintained.

A similar inverse relationship between social class and psychiatric disorder was found in the Midtown Study. The psychiatric protocols of the untreated persons revealed that the mental health "risk" of the lowest socioeconomic group was indeed greater than the "risk" for the middle and upper strata.[20] However, the "stresses" that the lower group encountered, as defined by the researchers, were not much greater than those encountered by people in the other two social strata. The researchers imply that those in the lower strata tend to react to stress more in terms of psychiatric symptoms than do those in the other status groupings.

Using an index of "mental health" in order to find the distribution of levels of psychological adjustment within a sample of Detroit automobile workers, Kornhauser[16] examined the distribution of mental health across several occupational groups. He found the lowest proportion of mentally healthy workers in the "repetitive, semiskilled" category in both young and middle-aged workers' groups. Assuming that these occupational categories are correlated with socioeconomic status, this study supports the hypothesis that the lower status groups show a lower proportion of mentally healthy individuals.

Gurin, Veroff, and Feld[11] have reported a study of the mental health of a national sample of the United States, in which they related their measures individually to education, income, and occupation. Again, analysis of the association between income and emotional adjustment showed the lowest social class grouping to score highest on the measures of anxiety or stress.

In a study of the psychological well-being of a sample of residents of four small Illinois communities, Bradburn and Caplovitz[3] found that the highest percentages of the "not too happy" were to be found among those with incomes of less than $3,000 and those with eighth-grade education or less. Furthermore, their measures of anxiety revealed that the highest proportion of those with high anxiety were among those with the least education.

Phillips[32] reported in his study of the prevalence of mental disorder in New Hampshire that education showed the most striking relationship to mental disorder. For example, almost 38 per cent of those with less than a high school education had scores of four or higher on the 22-Item Mental Health Scale[17] compared to about two per cent of those who were college graduates. None of the college graduates had scores indicating "severe" impairment (a score of 7 or higher), while 13.6 per cent of those who did not finish high school were found in that category.

Summarizing the results of these studies briefly, the subjects experiencing higher stress symptomatology or psychiatric impairment were found among those who had less income,[3] less formal education,[32] those whose husbands held lower occupational rank,[16] and those who could generally be characterized as members of lower socioeconomic strata.[11, 13, 20, 23, 40] These studies collectively and systematically reveal that members of lower socioeconomic groups have been found to be psychiatrically disturbed more frequently than have members of higher groups. These authors suggest that perhaps all of these factors reviewed above are part of a lower class life experience which results in a generalized lack of moral and social integration in a worthwhile group. In the following section, we review another suggestive line of research contained in some recent studies which look closely at the association between mental disturbance (as measured by the 22-Item Mental Health Scale developed by the Midtown researchers) and some general measures of adjustment to society among "normal" population samples.

Studies Concerned with the Relationship Between Psychiatric Impairment and General Measures of Adjustment

The first study to be considered here was concerned with deferment of gratification in a college setting. Among the hypotheses tested in this research was the following: "the greater the frequency of deferring social gratification, the poorer the student's mental health."[31] Based upon an examination of a random sample of 109 students constituting a systematic 4 per cent sample of the total student body at Dartmouth College, Phillips' data provided strong support for this hypothesis. The author concluded from his data that "students deferring gratification from social sources in order to realize academic gain do indeed realize more academic satisfaction while at the same time being discontent with their social life." Furthermore, the data supported Phillips' observation that: "Those deferring social gratification seem to end up being worse off than the nondeferrers; they not only are less socially satisfied but, in addition, have poorer mental health."[31] It thus appeared reasonable for the researcher to assume, as he did, that:

Lack of satisfactory involvement in the social life of the campus probably also means a lessened amount of contact with potential sources of support. For instance, the individual who frequently defers gratification from social sources in order to study for his classes will be unlikely to have much opportunity to discuss with his peers the gripes and dissatisfactions arising from the college environment. Even if he is no more dissatisfied with his situation than his non-deferring peers, he will have less chance to vent any of his dissatisfactions through bull-sessions and informal get-togethers. Thus, he may very well feel frustrated and unhappy with his situation [p. 337].

Most salient in the present context was the finding that individuals who deferred gaining the gratifications derived from social interaction were not only less socially satisfied but had poorer mental health; particularly was this true for those who had deferred for the longest period of time.

Pursuing the forgoing research further, Segal and Phillips[36] questioned whether their prior findings could possibly be the result of emotional disturbance which might conceivably have already been present among certain students at the time these students entered college. In other words, they wished to learn whether "it is more reasonable to view emotional disturbance in adolescents as a fixed condition affecting reactions to a specific social milieu, or whether, on the contrary, the choice of one pattern of behavior over another in that milieu is more likely to lead to subsequent disturbance."[36]

Summarizing briefly, this study showed that: (1) the initial emotional status of the students (determined by the Minnesota Multiphasic Personality Inventory administered at the time of college matriculation) exercised no appreciable determinative effects over whether or not students will be deferrers; (2) deferral and previous disturbance *both* affect current emotional status, but the effects of the former are, if anything, stronger than those of the latter; and (3) the negative impact of deferral occurs among both the initially disturbed and the initially healthy students. Furthermore, previously disturbed students become emotionally healthier through putting aside their work and sharing their leisure with their fellows.

In this study, Segal and Phillips demonstrated that the current emotional status of college students depends as much on participation in leisure activities (assumed to be stress-relieving) as it does on the mental health or disturbance of students upon their entrance to college. A reasonable interpretation of the findings of these two studies[31, 36] aggrees with Bradburn's observation[2] that: "The suggestion that factors which interfere with . . . the person's sense of membership in a definite human group and in a moral order are contributing causes of mental disturbance opens up new avenues of inquiry that have been severely neglected by researchers in the field of mental health."

Extending the work of Bradburn and his associates at the National Opinion Research Center,[3] Derek Phillips' research dealing with social participation and happiness carries forth the investigation of environmental factors and mental health or disturbance among nonhospitalized, "normal" populations. Basing his research squarely upon sociological theory, Phillips[33] points out that:

> Social participation has long been considered important as an index of social integration, reflecting common prescriptions and proscriptions for conduct and beliefs among individuals. Durkheim and Toennies, among others, were of course concerned with these aspects of social participation. Very little direct attention, however, has been given to empirical examinations of the consequences of social participation for a person's feelings of well-being or happiness [p. 480].

Happiness, according to Bradburn and his associates, is best conceptualized as a function of the relationship between two independent dimensions of (a) positive and (b) negative affect. Their findings have shown that positive and negative affect do not occupy two polar positions on a single dimension, but are two

192

separate dimensions which vary independently of one another. Employing a ten-item questionnaire containing items referring to five negative and five positive feelings, the researchers concluded that the difference between the scores on the positive and negative feelings indexes—which they call the Affect Balance Score—is a good indicator of an individual's current level of happiness.

In order to examine the relationship between voluntary social participation and self-reports of happiness, Phillips formulated three hypotheses: (1) the number of positive feelings which individuals experience is related to their voluntary social participation: the higher the extent of social participation, the greater the number of positive feelings they will report; (2) the number of negative feelings which individuals experience is not related to their voluntary social participation; and (3) happiness is related to social participation: the higher the extent of voluntary social participation, the greater the degree of happiness reported. The index of social participation used was composed of three measures: (1) the amount of contact with friends, (2) the number of neighbors known, and (3) the amount of organizational activity.

Analysis of the data provided strong support for all three hypotheses. Among the insights provided by this study was the finding that contacts with friends tended to increase the subjects' positive feelings to a greater extent than did either of the other types of social participation (that is, number of neighbors known or amount of organizational activity). In regard to this finding, Phillips[33] commented that:

A similar finding is reported by Langner and his associates on the Midtown Study Staff. Concerned with the relationship of mental illness to "Interpersonal Affiliation," they found that having no friends involved a greater risk of mental illness than did either lack of organizational activity or lack of visiting with neighbors [pp. 482, 483].

Another important disclosure of this investigation was the discovery of a very strong association existing between level of education and social participation. Phillips pointed out that:

Almost 54 per cent of those with college training were high on the social participation index, compared to 43.5 per cent of the high school graduates and 29.3 per cent of those with less than a high school education. This finding is in line with previous results and suggests that increased education tends to teach individuals more of the skills that facilitate participation, as well as enhancing their prestige and making them more desirable participants from the point of view of others [p. 487].

Continuing this line of inquiry in a subsequent study, Phillips was concerned with ascertaining the consequences of social participation for the happiness experienced by: (1) a group of individuals manifesting a high number of psychiatric symptoms, and (2) a group of individuals who are relatively symptom-free. Again, Phillips employed the 22-Item Mental Health Scale to measure mental health status; three variables—contact with friends, number of neighbors known, and organizational activity in addition to a composite index of the three—were used to measure subjects' degree of social participation. Degree of happiness was assessed by the subjects' self-reports concerning whether they were "very happy," "pretty happy," or "not too happy."

Both mental health status and social participation were employed as explanatory variables in relation to happiness. The data disclosed the following important findings: (1) subjects classified as mentally ill experienced a great deal less happiness than did those categorized as well and the relation between classification as ill or well and happiness was always maintained; (2) among both the ill and the well, the greater the social participation, the greater the percentage of respondents who report themselves as being "very happy"; and (3) for each of the three measures of social participation, mentally ill individuals who are high in participation are as happy or happier than well persons who are low in participation. Social participation and mental health status both, therefore, affect happiness independently of one another, supporting the hypothesis guiding this research.

Among the observations made by Phillips are the following: (1) that although both social participation and mental health status exert an independent influence on happiness, neither individually nor in combined form do the indicators of social participation exercise as much effect as mental health status; and (2) that it appears that mental health status precedes social participation in temporal sequence.

In drawing some conclusions from this study, Phillips[33] noted that:

Although social participation by itself appears to have a positive influence on the happiness people feel, it is considered important mainly as an indicator of positive feelings which derive from social intercourse . . . . Frequently, social contacts are intrinsically rewarding and serve as evidence of an individual's ability to establish satisfactory relationships with others. Our analyses here have shown that a high rate of social participation is associated with a relatively high level of happiness, even when an individual manifests a high number of psychiatric symptoms. Apparently, the therapeutic consequences of social participation help to some extent in counterbalancing the negative effects of mental illness [p. 290].

The foregoing research has important implications with regard to the ameliorative influence which interpersonal affiliation or meaningful supportive social involvement has in affecting the mental health status of the groups under investigation.

Deferment of gratification from social sources[31] by college students resulted not only in significantly reduced social satisfaction but also contributed to their poorer level of mental health. Examining the data on the Dartmouth sample in a more detailed analysis, the researchers[36] highlighted an even more serious impact of deferring gratification, in that doing so resulted in negative consequences for the mental health status of both initially disturbed and initially emotionally healthy students. These two studies demonstrate rather forcefully the importance which membership in a supportive peer group of students has for the mental health of these individuals.

Further evidence for the general finding relating to the importance of voluntary social participation, as an index of individual social integration, is found in Phillips' study of the effects of social participation on self-reports of happiness.[33] Not only were self-reports of happiness lightly related to social participation but the data revealed that the greater the extent of participation, the greater the degree of happiness reported by the respondents.

When both mental health status and social participation are employed as explanatory variables in relation to happiness,[31] the results further highlight "the ameliorative consequences of social participation as they affect the happiness experienced by the mentally ill."

These two studies[31] contain some important implications for the willingness of mentally ill persons to seek psychiatric assistance. For, as true prevalence studies have shown,[20,23,32,40] the greater majority of individuals classified as mentally ill have never sought psychiatric assistance for their illnesses. In regard to this finding, Phillips conjectures that: "Perhaps social participation has the effect of protecting people from having to seek psychiatric help because the positive feelings associated with participation tend to offset the unpleasurable feelings of psychiatric disorders."

The foregoing studies provide considerable support for the importance of social integration and the individual's feeling of being a significant part of a stable moral order in the community. This being the case, it is of considerable importance to investigate the effect which feelings of anomia, which interfere with the individual's sense of membership in the moral order, may have on the mental health status of members of various socioeconomic groups. For example, one might expect members of lower class standing to express a sense of anomia, but, as noted previously,[10] virtually no studies exist which link such social-psychological variables to psychiatric impairment when controlling for social class factors. The authors believe that anomia may be one of the variables influencing the development of emotional disorder regardless of class membership. The present investigation raises the question as to what it is about social classes that accounts for this relationship and whether or not feelings of anomia generated in a lower class milieu may not constitute an intervening variable between social class and mental health. In other words, we emphasize the need for specifying the social-psychological processes by which social class differences in feelings of anomia are subsequently translated into emotional well-being or illness. It seems reasonable to assume that most social factors which help explain the association between social class and psychiatric disorder can probably be understood as an increased sense of anomia resulting from nonintegration in a stable social order.

The implications for the mental health of the individuals lacking a sense of membership in the moral order (anomia) which were inherent, albeit from a positive viewpoint, in Phillips' studies are further investigated in a study of the prevalence of psychiatric impairment in a Western state.

Interrelations Between Anomia, Social Class, and Psychiatric Impairment

For a considerable length of time, sociologists have been concerned with the notion of anomie. As McClosky and Schaar[27] have noted: "Since Merton's seminal contribution of 1938, around 35 scientific papers have appeared on the subject of anomy most of them since 1950." As Durkheim[8] used the term, "anomie," it referred to the qualities of a group or the social structure and not to the characteristics of individuals. In a similar vein, Robert Merton[29] indicated that his theory referred to the cultural structure, on the one hand, and the social structure, on the other.

The terms "anomia" or "anomy" have come into current usage due to the need to focus upon the individual or psychological rather than the collective aspects of anomie. This psychological conception of anomia has been developed by Robert MacIver[24] and Leo Srole,[39] among others. To MacIver anomy meant a "state of mind in which the individual's sense of social cohesion—the mainspring of his morale—is broken or fatally weakened." Following soon after MacIver's work, Leo Srole developed a scale to measure anomia as the individual subjectively experiences it. This scale is made up of five items which purport to measure the individual's perception of his social environment and his place in it.

Because of the nature of the variables, anomia and psychiatric impairment, we believe it of importance to specify clearly the meaning of anomia as employed here as distinct from the connotation of personal alienation which is frequently used as a coping mechanism by persons having personal problems. Clinard[42] has provided a useful starting point with his insightful observation that anomia as used in the social psychological perspective refers, in part, to the subjective aspects of what Merton called anomie. The distinction is not always precise, but the alienated individual is considered marginal, normless, and isolated. This usage is similar to the meaning implied in the concept by Srole,[39] Meier and Bell,[28] and others. The individual is considered alienated from society, but this is not the same as personal disorganization or psychiatric impairment. We are in agreement with Nettler,[30] who has pointed out that the concepts anomia and alienation should:

> . . . [not] be equated, as they so often are, with personal disorganization defined as intrapersonal disorganization, conflict, personal goallessness, or lack of "internal coherence," and which is used synonymously with

196

psychopathology. Behaviors commonly selected as symptoms of anomie such as white collar crime or juvenile gang activity are often exhibited by individuals who are themselves well integrated. How alienated such people feel, as compared with those whose behaviors seem less indicative of anomie, is a matter for investigation rather than assumption. Similarly one may conceivably be alienated with or without personal disorganization and with or without participating in behaviors that are ordinarily used as indices for anomie [p. 672].

McClosky and Schaar,[27] in an insightful paper which parallels Nettler's thinking, conceptualize anomia as a state of mind, "a cluster of attitudes, beliefs, and feelings in the minds of individuals. Specifically, it is the feeling that the world and oneself are adrift, wandering, lacking in clear rules and stable moorings." Their theory clearly links anomic feelings with lower social status, as follows:

. . . those who occupy social positions remote from the mainstream exhibit a high incidence and intensity of anomic feelings. Because of poverty, or little education, these people are relatively isolated from the cultural mainstream. This condition reduces communication and impairs their ability to learn the norms of the larger community which, in turn, gives rise to feelings of normlessness [p. 20].

One area of an individual's life functioning in which one might reasonably expect the influence of mental health or disturbance to be felt is in the degree to which he feels himself to be a significant part of a moral order and a stable societal network (in other words, the extent to which he feels integrated or nonanomic). On the other hand, by implication, the individual who reports himself not to be experiencing anomia would be expected to have better mental health than the individual who feels anomic. It would seem consistent with the suggestion of Davis[5] that relationships among various types of subjective (self-rating) measures of mental health (and other social psychological measures such as anomia) are particularly important because a case can be made for their face validity. That is, while a person who thinks he has a heart condition may or may not have one, anyone who reports feeling anomic really does feel that "the world and (himself) are adrift, wandering, lacking in clear rules and stable moorings. The anomic feels literally demoralized; for him, the norms governing behavior are weak, ambiguous, and remote. He lives in a normative 'low pressure' area, a turbulent region of weak and fitful currents of moral meaning. The core of the concept is the feeling of moral emptiness."[27]

The major premise underlying the present research is that anomia, conceptualized as including feelings of demoralization which reflect the individual's lack of a sense of membership in the moral order, is characteristic of lower socioeconomic groups. Furthermore, we assume that anomic feelings are associated with the development and expression of symptoms indicative of psychiatric impairment. This conceptualization follows Srole's[38, 39] reformulation of anomia as including both psychological as well as sociological processes.

Because a sizeable proportion of individuals of lower social class standing have less education, lower ranking occupations, and less access to societal resources,[6, 15, 20, 27, 34] a parallel assumption, consistent with Srole's findings, is that a higher proportion of these individuals tend to feel more anomic and consequently experience higher rates of psychiatric symptomatology. As such, our assumption is that this is one reason why a higher proportion of persons with psychiatric impairments are found in lower socioeconomic groups.

The present investigation then attempts to further clarify the interrelationships between social class and anomia variables as these are related to mental disorder.[43] The assumption is tested that psychiatric symptomatology is a response to stress of a type more often experienced by anomic persons than by nonanomics in the community irrespective of social class membership. Furthermore, we would expect that persons experiencing feelings of anomia in each of the social classes would report high psychiatric symptomatology when compared with persons not experiencing feelings of anomia.

Our final assumption is that a greater proportion of persons in lower socioeconomic status groups would experience psychiatric impairments because a larger percentage of these individuals are anomic. In sum, we are not postulating a one-to-one relationship between anomia and psychiatric impairment; rather, we are arguing that anomia may be one of a number of factors contributing to psychiatric impairment and, as such, the higher an individual's level of anomia, the greater will be the probability of the subject expressing symptoms indicative of psychiatric impairment regardless of social class standing.

An examination of these assumptions was made by testing the following hypotheses:

Hypothesis I: Subject's socioeconomic status (as determined by indices of formal education, husband's occupation, and social class position) will be significantly associated with level of psychiatric impairment.

Hypothesis II: Subject's level of anomia will be significantly related to the subject's psychiatric symptom level.

Hypothesis III: Subject's feelings (or level) of anomia will maintain a significant relationship with subject's psychiatric symptom level within each socioeconomic status category investigated.

Methods

The study population was made up of mothers of families with children under five years of age residing in a Western state. The subjects (n = 916) were selected by the use of a two-stage probability sampling technique.[37] The data for this study were drawn from interviews with the subjects in their homes. Level of anomia was measured by the Srole scale.[39]

Socioeconomic status was determined by using Hollingshead's[12] *Two-Factor Index of Social Position*. In addition, two commonly used measures of socioeconomic status—subject's formal education and husband's occupational rank—were employed. Occupational ranking of subject's husband was determined through the use of Warner's[41] categories of occupational ranking. Subject's level of formal education was dichotomized into two categories: persons having completed high school only and those having 13 or more years of formal education.

Psychiatric impairment was determined on the basis of subjects' responses to the 22-Item Mental Health Scale developed by the Midtown Manhattan Project staff.[17] This scale yields a score which predicts the probability of an individual being labelled as psychiatrically impaired were he to be interviewed by a psychiatrist. Two different validity studies of this instrument document that it is adequate for screening and case-finding in large populations and that the probability of psychiatric impairment increases as the scores run higher.[17,25] Following Langner, a cut-off point of 4 was used to categorize subjects with scores above this point as experiencing psychiatric impairment, while subjects with scores below this point were considered to have average or good mental health. In validating the scale, Langner and his associates found that a score of 4 or higher indicated "serious" psychiatric impairment.[17, 20] On the other hand, of the people classified as "well" by the Midtown study psychiatrists, only 1 per cent had scores of 4 or more; but among those classified as "incapacitated" (serious symptoms with great and total impairment), 84 per cent had a score of 4 or more.*

Statistical analysis. The Mantel-Haenszel procedure[26] corrected for continuity was used to test the significance of the association of anomia and psychiatric impairment. This procedure yields a 1 degree of freedom chi-square. The scores used in the procedure were 0, 1, . . . and following Mantel's suggestion a continuity correction of 1/2 was used, that is, 1/2 the smallest difference between adjacent scores.

In addition, the statistic R (estimated relative risk) was used.[4] This is a ratio of the proportion of subjects experiencing psychiatric symptoms for those who have a factor (anomia, low socioeconomic status, and so forth) divided by the ratio of

---

*The importance of the 22-Item Screening Score as a research instrument for measuring psychiatric impairment is attested to by the following group of studies in which it has been used: Phillips; [31] [32] [33] Segal and Phillips;[36] Manis, and his associates[25] Langner;[19] Blumenthal;[1] Dohrenwend;[6] Fabrega and his coworkers.[9]

the proportion for those who do not have the factor. The ratio of proportions was used instead of estimated odds (often also called "relative risk") because a population sample was obtained which allowed estimation of proportions which are not available in the usual retrospective studies.

Findings

We turn first to a presentation of data related to our first hypothesis (Table I). When we consider amount of formal education, we find that 16 per cent of our subjects who had completed 13 or more years of education reported mental disturbance; while that percentage was more than doubled (36.0 per cent) among respondents who had completed only high school or less. If we examine the

TABLE 1 — Per Cent High (4+) Psychiatric Symptom Level, Relative Risk, Chi-Square and P by Formal Education, Husband's Occupation and Socioeconomic Status Categories

Variables	Per cent High (4+) Psychiatric Symptom Level	R+	X^{2*}	P
FORMAL EDUCATION				
13+ years	16.3	0.45		
	$(n=233)^a$			
0-12 years	36.0	2.21		
	$(n=683)$		30.60	.0001
HUSBAND'S OCCUPATION				
Professional & Semi-Professional	18.0	0.54		
	$(n=183)$			
Clerks & Kindred Workers	28.8	0.92		
	$(n=326)$			
Skilled & Semi-Skilled	38.1	1.53		
	$(n=357)$		23.06	.0001
SOCIOECONOMIC STATUS				
I-II	17.5	0.53		
	$(n=154)$			
III	24.3	0.74		
	$(n=226)$			
IV	33.5	1.18		
	$(n=376)$			
V	47.8	1.74		
	$(n=134)$		34.82	.0001

[a] Figures in parentheses are base for percentages.

R + = Relative Risk, compared to *all others* not in the category (computed by the ratio of proportions, not estimated odds.)

*All X²s (1 d.f.) corrected for continuity, obtained by the Mantel-Haenszel Procedure.
Reprinted with permission from "Behavioral Publications," New York.

200

relative risk associated with these two educational categories ($R = 2.21$ and $R = 0.45$), we find that the estimated probability is over twice as great that subjects with less education (0 to 12 years) will experience mental disturbance (as measured by number of symptoms reported) compared with respondents who have 13 or more years of education. The Mantel-Haenszel X^2 (30.60) is highly statistically significant, and these findings confirm our first hypothesis in terms of subject's formal education.

When the data are categorized by a second index of socioeconomic status (husband's occupation), the findings disclose that 38 per cent of the subjects with husbands in skilled or semi-skilled jobs reported mental disturbance; while less than one-half that percentage was found among wives of professional or semi-professional men (18.0 per cent). Comparing each category with all other categories, one finds a progression of increasing relative risk: $R = 0.54$, $R = 0.92$, and $R = 1.53$. These data reveal that the estimated probability is over one and one-half times as great for subjects married to men in the skilled, semi-skilled category as compared to subjects married to men in higher occupational groupings, to report high psychiatric symptomatology.

The last observation to be made about Table 1 is concerned with the grouping of subjects into social classes. This was calculated by the use of the Hollingshead Two-Factor Index of Social Class Position and based upon husband's education and occupation. In this analysis, we find that 17 per cent of the subjects in Classes I-II report high psychiatric symptomatology; while this percentage is almost three times as great (47.8 per cent) among Class V respondents. Comparing each category with all other categories as one proceeds from Classes I-II through Class V, we again find a progression of increasing relative risk: $R = 0.53$, $R = 0.74$, $R = 1.18$, and $R = 1.74$. Thus, we find that the estimated probability is one and three-quarter times as great that members of Class V will experience mental disturbance when compared with members of other Classes. In summary, the three indices of socioeconomic status all provide strong, statistically significant, support for our first hypothesis.

Analysis relative to the second hypothesis that anomia will be significantly related to subject's psychiatric symptomatology is presented in Table 2. These data reveal that the proportion of subjects with high levels of psychiatric impairment in the high anomia group is two times that for the low anomia group ($R = 2.00$). Relative risk indicates that the estimated probability is twice as great that highly anomic subjects will report high psychiatric symptom levels as the probability that low anomic respondents will report such disturbance. Of the group with high anomia, 40 per cent experienced mental disturbance, while the percentage of mental disturbance was only half that great (20.0 per cent) in the group of low anomia respondents. These data clearly support our second hypothesis.

Findings relative to our third hypothesis are presented in Table 3. These data disclose that among subjects with 13 or more years of education, only 8.9 per cent with low anomia appear to have some form of psychiatric impairment; whereas 28.7 per cent of the highly anomic group report psychiatrically impairing

TABLE 2 — Per Cent Reporting Low and High Psychiatric Symptom Levels by Anomia Score.

Anomia Score	Subjects' Psychiatric Symptom Level		Total
	0 - 3	4+	
Low Anomia	80.0	20.0	100.0
	(n=324) [a]	(n=81)	(n=405)
High Anomia	60.1	39.9	100.0
	(n=307)	(n=204)	(n=511)
Total	68.9	31.1	100.0
	(n=631)	(n=285)	(n=916)

X^2 = 40.86,[b] (1 d.f.), P<.0001 corrected for continuity, computed by the Mantel-Haenszel Procedure.

R = 2.00 (The relative risk computed by the ratio of proportions, not estimated odds.)

[a] Figures in parentheses are actual frequencies

[b] Because none of the socioeconomic variables were controlled, the X^2 = 40.86 is biased; when it is controlled for socioeconomic status in four categories the summary X^2 = 28.61 and hence is still highly statistically significant.

symptoms. Relative risk (R = 3.22) indicates that in this group the estimated probability is over three times as great that highly anomic respondents will report a high number of symptoms as the probability that low anomic respondents will report such symptoms. Respective X^2 values (X^2 = 14.23 and X^2 = 16.56) are highly statistically significant.

When the husband's occupational ranking is held constant, we find that among those women whose husbands are professionals or semi-professionals, only 7 per cent with low anomia report high psychiatric symptomatology; while 37 per cent of those with high anomia report mental disturbance. The relative risk (R = 5.26) discloses that the estimated probability is five and one-quarter times as great that subjects who feel highly anomic will report a high number of psychiatric symptoms as the probability that low anomic subjects will report such symptoms. Among subjects married to clerks and kindred workers, the association between anomia and psychiatric symptom level was positive (R = 1.39) and, although not statistically significant at the .05 level, a trend of association was clearly indicated (P = .080).

The findings in Table 3 further reveal that among members of Socioeconomic Classes I-II, 8 per cent of the subjects with low anomia report mental disturbance, while over 34 per cent with high anomia report such impairment. It is of interest to compare these percentages with those for Class V respondents, where 34 per cent of the subjects with low anomia report high psychiatric symptoms and over 54 per cent with high anomia experienced such impairment. A comparison of relative risks for these categories is of interest (R = 4.21 and R = 1.60). Among members of Classes I-II, the relative risk indicates that the esti-

TABLE 3 — Per Cent High (4+) Psychiatric Symptom Level of High Anomic and Low Anomic Subjects, Relative Risk, Chi-Square and P, by Formal Education, Husband's Occupation and Socioeconomic Status Categories.

Control Variables	Per cent High Psychiatric Symptom Level		$R+$	X^2*	P
	High Anomia	Low Anomia			
FORMAL EDUCATION					
13+ years	28.7	8.9	3.22	14.23	.0002
(n = 233)	(n = 87)[a]	(n = 146)			
0-12 years	42.0	26.3	1.59	16.56	.0001
(n = 683)	(n = 424)	(n = 259)			
HUSBAND'S OCCUPATION					
Professional & Semi-Professional	36.8	7.0	5.26	23.58	.0001
(n = 183)	(n = 68)	(n = 115)			
Clerks & Kindred Workers	33.3	23.9	1.39	3.09	.080
(n = 326)	(n = 171)	(n = 155)			
Skilled & Semi-Skilled	43.5	27.1	1.61	8.30	.004
(n = 357)	(n = 239)	(n = 118)			
SOCIOECONOMIC STATUS					
I-II	34.5	8.2	4.21	15.00	.0001
(n = 153)	(n = 55)	(n = 98)			
III	32.2	16.2	1.99	6.94	.008
(n = 226)	(n = 115)	(n = 111)			
IV	38.5	25.9	1.49	5.76	.017
(n = 374)	(n = 231)	(n = 143)			
V	54.4	34.1	1.60	4.09	.043
(n = 134)	(n = 90)	(n = 44)			

[a] Base for percentages.

$R+$ = Relative Risk (computed by the ratio of proportions, not estimated odds.)

*All X^2s (1 d.f.) corrected for continuity, obtained by the Mantel-Haenszel Procedure.

mated probability is over four times as great that subjects who are highly anomic will report mental disturbance as the probability that low anomic respondents will do so. On the other hand, among Class V respondents, the estimated probability (R = 1.60), is only one and one-half times as great that highly anomic subjects will report high symptom levels as is the probability that low anomic respondents will so report. Chi-square values are significant at the .04 level or less.

These findings lead to the acceptance of the third study hypothesis which stated that a significant relationship would be found to persist between anomia and mental disturbance within each education, occupation, and social class grouping investigated. Furthermore, going beyond a simple consideration of the magnitude of the percentage who are psychiatrically impaired within each social status category, we begin to see the noteworthy meaning of these differences by employing a comparison of the relative risk of psychiatric impairment among the anomic versus the nonanomic within each category. Using percentage comparisons (Table 3), we see that the proportion impaired for both high and low anomic persons varies directly with socioeconomic status variables. For instance, the percentage with high psychiatric symptom levels among highly anomic persons with 0 to 12 years of education was 42 per cent compared to 29 per cent for highly anomic persons with 13 or more years of education. However, looking within each educational grouping, one finds that the *relative risk* (R = 3.22) of experiencing high psychiatric symptomatology in the high-education, high-anomic group compared to the high-education, low-anomic group is *greater* than that for the low-education, high-anomic group compared to the low-education, low-anomic group (R = 1.59). Similar findings occur for the two other ways of socioeconomic classification given in Table 3. In summary, one may conclude that despite decreased proportions of persons with psychiatric impairment within the high social status categories, the presence or absence of anomia is *more critical for persons with high, rather than low, social class standing.*

SUMMARY AND IMPLICATIONS

This chapter represents an effort to investigate anomia as one social psychological variable intervening between social class factors and psychiatric impairment and thus provide clues to the dynamic process underlying the relationship between social class standing and psychiatric disorder among normal populations. A number of studies have provided substantive evidence that the lowest classes have the highest rates of psychiatric impairment in our society.[3,11,13,16,20,23,31,40] The present investigation extends and further specifies two prior findings from the Midtown Manhattan Study which indicated that both socioeconomic status and anomia were associated with mental disturbance.[38,40]

Employing a broad theoretical interpretation of anomia, incorporating the insights of Srole,[38,39] and McClosky and Schaar[27] among others, we characterized the anomic individual as one who feels "literally demoralized . . . feeling that the world and himself are adrift, wandering, lacking in clear rules and stable moorings."[27] Furthermore, the highly anomic individual lacks a sense of social integration; he lacks a feeling of membership in a definite human group and in a moral order, which results in a personality exhibiting less resilience to withstand changing demands.

Further evidence of the crucial importance for mental health of a sense of integration with a significant reference group was found in a group of studies which focused on the association between mental disturbance and a number of general measures of adjustment to society, such as social participation, social satisfaction, and happiness. These studies collectively provided support for the notion, albeit from a slightly different perspective, that integration with significant reference groups from which the person gains meaningful involvement has a crucial and positive influence upon individual mental health. In fact, meaningful social participation was thought to have "the effect of protecting people from having to seek psychiatric help because the positive feelings associated with participation tend to offset the unpleasureable feelings of psychiatric disorders."[33]

Finally, the chapter focused upon our study concerning the interrelationships between anomia, socioeconomic status, and mental disturbance. Summarizing briefly, the findings revealed that both socioeconomic status and anomia are associated with psychiatric impairment. Not only were these results confirmed but anomia was found to maintain a significant relationship with psychiatric impairment within each education, occupation, and socioeconomic status grouping investigated.

Of particular interest was the fact that the proportion of subjects reporting psychiatric symptomatology *decreases* with *increasing* status, but that the *relative risk* of such symptoms for highly anomic persons (compared to nonanomic subjects within each status grouping) is *much higher for the highest status groups than for the lower groups.*

One suggested interpretation of these findings, consistent with social psychological theory, is that meanings are largely situational in nature and that the high status individual, if anomic, will more likely respond by experiencing mental disturbance than will lower class persons, who more frequently feel anomic, are surrounded by others who are anomic, that is, live in a contextually consonant environment.[35] On the other hand, the high status individual, if anomic, differs from his peers in this psychosocial attitude, that is, he will live in a contextually dissonant environment, and, we hypothesize, is more likely to respond by developing symptoms of psychiatric impairment.

The major contribution of the present investigation is an attempt to clarify the dynamic processes underlying the strong inverse relationship between social class standing and psychiatric impairment which has been so clearly evidenced in numerous prior research findings. Because there has been virtually no effort to study the complex processes underlying this relationship,[10] the present research was designed to examine anomia as one social psychological variable which intervenes between social class factors and psychiatric impairment. Our findings have provided clear support for the notion that anomia or the lack of integration with significant reference groups is indeed one factor linking social class standing and psychiatric impairment. The literature review and findings presented in this chapter should point toward further research on anomia and other social and psychological variables which may intervene between social class standing and psychiatric impairment.

REFERENCES

1. BLUMETHAL, M.D.: "Mental Health Among the Divorced: A Field Study of Divorced and Never Divorced Persons. *Archives of General Psychiatry* 16:603-608, 1967.
2. BRADBURN, N.M.: Review of Dorothea C. Leighton, et al., *The Character of Danger.* *American Journal of Sociology* 71:343, 1965.

3. BRADBURN, N.M., AND CAPLOVITZ, D.: *Reports on Happiness: A Pilot Study of Behavior Related to Mental Health.* Chicago: Aldine, 1965.

4. CHASE, G., AND KLAUBER, M.: "A Graph of Sample Sizes for Retrospective Studies." *American Journal of Public Health* 55:1993-1996, 1965.

5. DAVIS, J.A.: *Education for Positive Mental Health.* Chicago: Aldine, 1965.

6. DOHRENWEND, B.P.: "Social Status and Psychological Disorder: An Issue of Substance and an Issue of Method." *American Sociological Review* 31:14-34, 1966.

7. DOHRENWEND, B.P., AND DOHRENWEND, B.S.: *Social Status and Psychological Disorder: A Causal Inquiry.* New York, John Wiley, 1969.

8. DURKHEIM, E.: Le Suicide. Paris: Alcan. English Edition: *Suicide: A Study in Sociology.* Translated by John A. Spaulding and George Simpson. Glencoe, Ill.: The Free Press, 1951, 1897.

9. FABREGA, H., RUBEL, A.J., AND WALLACE, C.A.: "Working Class Mexican Psychiatric Outpatients." *Archives of General Psychiatry* 16:704-712, 1967.

10. FRIED, M.: "Social Differences in Mental Health," in John Kosa, Aaron Antonovsky and Irving K. Zola (eds.): *Poverty and Health: A Sociological Analysis.* Cambridge: Harvard University Press, Pp. 113-167, 1969.

11. GURIN, G., VEROFF, J., AND FELD, S.: *Americans View Their Mental Health.* New York: Basic Books, 1960.

12. HOLLINGSHEAD, A.B.: *Two Factor Index of Social Position.* New Haven: Privately mimeographed, 1957.

13. HOLLINGSHEAD, A.B., AND REDLICH, F.C.: *Social Class and Mental Illness:* A Community Study, New York: John Wiley, 1958.

14. HUGHES, C.C., TREMBLAY, M.A., RAPOPORT, R.N., AND LEIGHTON, A.H.: *People of Cove and Woodlot: Communities from the Viewpoint of Social Psychiatry,* Volume 2. New York: Basic Books, 1960.

15. IRELAN, L.M. (ed.): *Low-Income Life Styles.* Washington, D.C.: United States Government Printing Office, 1966.

16. KORNHAUSER, A.: *Mental Health of the Industrial Worker.* New York: John Wiley, 1965.

17. LANGNER, T.S.: "A Twenty-Two Item Screening Score of Psychiatric Symptoms Indicating Impairment." *Journal of Health and Human Behavior* 3:269-276, 1962.

18. LANGNER, T.S.: "Environmental Stress and Mental Health," in Paul H. Hoch and Joseph Zubin (eds.): *Comparative Epidemiology of the Mental Disorders.* New York: Grune & Stratton, 1961, pp. 32-44.

19. LANGNER, T.S.: "Psychophysiological Symptoms and the Status of Women in Two Mexican Communities," in Jane M. Murphy and Alexander H. Leighton (eds.): *Approaches to Cross-Cultural Psychiatry.* Ithaca, New York: Cornell University Press, 1965.

20. LANGNER, T.S., AND MICHAEL, S.T.: *Life Stress and Mental Health: The Midtown Manhattan Study,* Volume 2. New York: The Free Press, 1963.

21. LEIGHTON, A.H.: *My Name is Legion: Foundations for a Theory of Man in Relation to Culture,* Volume 1. New York: Basic Books, 1959.

22. LEIGHTON, D.C., HARDING, J.S., MACKLIN, D.B., HUGHES, C.C., AND LEIGHTON, A.H.: "Psychiatric findings of the Stirling County Study." *American Journal of Psychiatry* 119:1021-1026, 1963.

23. LEIGHTON, D.C., HARDING, J.S., MACKLIN, D.B., MACMILLAN, A.M., AND LEIGHTON, A.H.: *The Character of Danger: Psychiatric Symptoms in Selected Communities,* Volume 3. New York: Basic Books, 1963.

24. MacIVER, R.M.: *The Ramparts We Guard.* New York: The Macmillan Company, 1950.

25. MANIS, J.G., BRAWER, M.J., HUNT, C.L., AND KERCHER, L.: "Estimating the Prevalence of Mental Illness." *American Sociological Review* 29:84-89, 1964.

26. MANTEL, N.: "Chi-Square Tests with One Degree of Freedom: Extensions of the Mantel-Haenszel Procedure." *Journal of the American Statistical Association* 58:690-700, 1963.

27. McCLOSKY, H., AND SCHAAR, J.H.: "Psychological Dimensions of Anomy." *American Sociological Review* 21:709-716, 1965.

28. MEIER, D.L., AND BELL, W.: "Anomia and Differential Access to the Achievement of Life Goals." *American Sociological Review* 24:189-208, 1959.

29. MERTON, R.K.: "Social Structure and Anomie." *Social Theory and Social Structure.* Glencoe, Ill.: The Free Press, 1957.

30. NETTLER, G.: "A Measure of Alienation." *American Sociological Review* 22:670-677, 1957.

31. PHILLIPS, D.L.: "Deferred Gratification in a College Setting: Some Costs and Gains." *Social Problems* 13:333-343, 1966.

32. PHILLIPS, D.L.: "The 'True' Prevalence of Mental Illness in a New England State." *Community Mental Health Journal* 2:35-40, 1966.

33. PHILLIPS, D.L.: "Mental Health Status, Social Participation and Happiness." *Journal of Health and Social Behavior* 8:285-291, 1967.

34. ROMAN, P.M., AND TRICE, H.M.: *Schizophrenia and the Poor.* Ithaca, New York: Cornell University Press, 1967.

35. ROSENBERG, M.: "The Dissonant Religious Context and Emotional Disturbance." *American Journal of Sociology* 68:1-10, 1962.

36. SEGAL, B.E., AND PHILLIPS, D.L.: "Work, Play, and Emotional Disturbance: An Examination of Environment and Disturbance." *Archives of General Psychiatry* 16:173-179, 1967.

37. SERFLING, R.E., AND SHERMAN, I.L.: Attribute Sampling Methods for Local Health Departments with Special Reference to Immunization Surveys. Washington, D.C.: United States Government Printing Office, 1965.

38. SROLE, L.: "Interdisciplinary Conceptualization and Research in Social Psychiatry." Unpublished paper read before the American Sociological Society, Detroit, 1956.

39. SROLE, L.: "Social Integration and Certain Corollaries: An Exploratory Study." *American Sociological Review* 21:709-716, 1956.

40. SROLE, L., LANGNER, T.S., MICHAEL, S.T., OPLER, M.K., AND RENNIE, T.A.C.: *Mental Health in the Metropolis: The Midtown Manhattan Study,* Volume 1. New York: McGraw-Hill, 1962.

41. WARNER, L., MEEKER, M., AND EELLS, K.: *Social Class in America.* Chicago: Science Research Associates, 1949.

42. CLINARD, M.B.: *Anomie and Deviant Behavior.* New York: The Free Press, 1964.

43. REINHARDT, A.M., AND GRAY, R.M.: "Anomia, Socioeconomic Status and Mental Disturbance." *Community Mental Health Journal* 8:109-119, 1972.

Index

ADMISSION, inpatient treatment, discharge and, 51-58

Adjustment, psychiatric impairment and, 191-196

Aggression, depression and, 142

Aging, Projective Biography Test and, 152, 153

Anglo-Saxon women, depression and, 149

Anomia
definition of, 196, 197
interrelations among social class, psychiatric impairment and 185-207
methods of measuring, 199
Midtown Manhattan Study, socioeconomic status and, 186-189
psychiatric impairment and, statistical analysis of, 199, 200

Anomie, suicide, Durkheim and, 161, 162

BEHAVIOR
cultural variations in patterns of, 99
depression and acculturated, 146

Black women, depression and, 149

Bureaucracy, model of, in mental illness, 52-54

CAREER
mental patient's
first stage, 45, 46
second stage, 46-50
third stage, 51-58

Chronicity, mental illness label and, 50

Class-Schizophrenia relationship, interpretation of, 121-123

Class social. See Social Class.

Cognitive dissonance, depression and, 142, 143

Community psychiatry, adjoining service areas in, 11-13

Conflict
cross-cultural research and interprofessional, 83
depression and ego, 142

Conformity, social class and, 129-131

Coroners, suicide rates and, 173

Cross-cultural research
availability of staff in, 81-83
classification of societies and, 89, 90
comparability of data in, 86-89
critical interviews and instrument construction versus surveys in, 86-89
cultural variations, psychiatric diagnosis and, 98-100
data collection in, 86-89
diagnostic problems of psychiatric disorder in, 98-100
differential distribution of social class and, 95, 96
epidemiological studies and, 91, 92
ethics in, 92, 93
interdependent collaboration and, 83-85
language barrier in, 85, 86
measurement and comparability of social class and mobility in, 93-100
methological problems in, 81-86, 89-93
migration and, 96, 97, 98
personal characteristics of interviewers in, 82, 83
problems in psychiatric sociology and, 81-103
problems with measurement of social class and, 93-97
psychiatric disorder, diagnostic problems and, 98-110
relationship between migration and mental illness in, 97, 98
sampling problems in, 89-92
social mobility, level of occupation and, 96, 97
stigma attached to mental illness and, 90-92
strategies and models of, 83-86
successive and concurrent methods of data collection and, 83-85

Cultural perception, suicide and, 179

Cultural variations, onset of schizophrenia, manic-depression and, 35-39

Culture
behavior patterns and variations in, 99
patient, mental illness and, 54-58

DATA
collection of
in cross-cultural research, 86-89
successive and concurrent methods in, 83-85
Durkheim, preconceived suicide theory and, 161

Data—*continued*
  incidence versus prevalence, in mental illness, 120, 121
Death, stigma and types of, 166-168
Depression
  aggression and, 142, 150
  Anglo-Saxon women and, 149
  as symptom choice, 146, 147
  Black women and, 149
  cognitive dissonance and, 142, 143
  ego-psychological theory of, 142
  ethnicity and influence on, 149-155
  existential approach to, 142, 143
  family identification and, 140, 141, 151
  hostility and, 142
  Jewish women and, 149, 151
  loss and, 142-144
  middle age and, 140, 143, 145-151
  neglect of, 139-142
  problems in studying, 141, 142
  role loss and, 147-155
  role theory and, 144-146
  social class and, 140, 141,
  sociological approach to, 144-147
  sympathy and, 146
  theoretical explanations for, 142-144
  women and, 140, 149
Diagnostic category, erratic nature of, 71, 72
Diagnostic problems, cross-cultural study of psychiatric disorder and, 98-100
Discharge, inpatient admission, treatment and, 51-58
Discrimination, mental disorder and lower-class, 122
Disordered behavior
  definition of, 25, 26
  personality traits and, 31
Drift hypothesis, schizophrenia and, 117-119
Durkheim
  suicide and, 160-164, 182
  social meanings of, 178, 179

Ecological fallacy, sociology, suicide, and, 163, 164
Education
  levels of
    psychiatric disorder and, 190
    social class and, 93
Ego conflict and depression, 142
Epidemiological studies, problems with, 91, 92
Epidemiology of psychiatric impairment in normal populations, 186-189
Ethics in cross-cultural research, 92, 93
Ethnicity
  depression and influence of, 149-155
  schizophrenia and, 122, 123
Existentialism, depression and, 142, 143

Family
  depression and identification with, 140, 141, 151
  history of psychiatric disorder and, 75, 76
  response to mental illness and, 46, 47
  social class, schizophrenia, and, 127-129
First career stage, mental patient and, 45, 46
Follow-up studies, social causes of psychiatric disorder and, 69-71

Genetic explanations, ruling out physical and, in psychiatric disorder, 75, 76
Genetics, schizophrenia, stress and, 123-125
Guilt, metadepression and, 140

High-risk populations, identifying and obtaining samples of, 70, 71
Hospital admission
  social class, schizophrenia, and, 120
  treatment and discharge and, 51-58
Hospitalization, mental disorder and lower-class, 122
Hostility, depression and, 142

Identity
  indices for schizophrenia, 120, 121
  involutional psychosis and loss of, 144, 145
  sociology and psychiatry, fusions and fissions of, 5-17
Inpatient admission, treatment and discharge, 51-58
Integration, sociological concern with lack of, 140
Interrelations among anomia, social class, and psychiatric impairment, 185-207
Interviewers, personal characteristics of, 82, 83
Interviews
  history of psychiatric disorder and, 73
  operation of social variables and, 77
Involutional psychosis, loss of identity and, 144, 145
Isolation, schizophrenia and, 34, 35, 123

Jewish women, depression and, 149, 151

Labeling, psychiatric referral and/or, 46-50
Labeling theory
  first career stage in, 45, 46
  mental illness and, 43-62
  patient culture and, 54-58
  second career stage in, 46-50
  third career stage in, 51-58
Language barrier in cross-cultural research, 85, 86
Loss, depression and, 142-144

Manic-depression, schizophrenia and, cultural variations in onset of, 35-39

210

Marital role loss, depression and, 149
Maternal role loss, depression and, 147, 149, 151, 152
Measurement, comparability and, of social class, 93-97
Mental disorder
  deferment of social gratification and, 191-195
  lower-class discrimination and, 122
Mental hospital, bureaucratic nature of, 52-54
Mental illness
  chronicity of label and, 50
  cultural variations in, symptoms of, 98-100
  family and, 46, 47
  first career stage of, 45, 46
  incidence versus prevalence of, data on, 120, 121
  labeling theory and, 43-62
    patient culture and, 54-58
  measuring social mobility and, 96, 97
  migration and, problems in studying relationship between, 97, 98
  model of bureaucracy in, 52-54
  occupation and, 115
  patient nonresponsibility and, 50
  prevasiveness of label and, 49, 50
  problems with epidemiological studies of, 91, 92
  search for causes of, 63-79
  second career stage of, 46-50
  sociopsychological role theory and, 44, 45
  stigma attached to, 89-92
  third career stage of, 51-58
  unclear scope and intent of institutional concept and, 51, 52
Metadepression, guilt and, 140
Methodological problems and cross-cultural research in psychiatric sociology, 81-86, 89-93
Middle age, depression and, 140, 143, 145-151
Midtown Manhattan Study
  analysis of social stability and, 30, 31
  socioeconomic status, anomia, and, 186-189
Migration, mental illness and, problems in studying relationship between, 97, 98
Models, strategies and, in cross-cultural research, 83-86
Motives, classification of, suicide and, 166, 175

Nonresponsibility, mental illness label and, 50
Normal, definition of, 185, 186

Occupation
  mental illness and, 115
  social class and, 94
  social mobility and level of, 96, 97
  women, depression and, 150, 152
Occupational mobility, social class, schizophrenia and, 116, 118, 119

Patient culture in mental illness, 54-58
Pervasiveness in mental illness label, 49, 50
Physical explanations, ruling out genetic and, in psychiatric disorder, 75, 76
Population(s)
  differential distribution of social class in, 95, 96
  epidemiology of psychiatric impairment in normal, 186-189
  identifying and obtaining samples of high-risk, 70, 71
  samples of, based on social variables predating psychiatric disorders, 68-78
  schizophrenia and urban, 115
Prelabeling, 45, 46
Problem-centered and theory-centered research, 31, 32
Problems of cross-cultural research in psychiatric sociology, 81-103
Projective Biography Test, aging and, 152, 153
Property, social class and influence of, 94
Psychiatric disorder
  bias created by duration of, 64, 65
  cross-cultural study of, 98-100
  educational levels and, 190
  equalizing time spans for, 74, 75
  family history of, 75, 76
  follow-up studies and social causes of, 69-71
  informants, records and, 69, 70, 73, 74
  interviews and history of, 73
  obtaining estimates for development of, 71-74
  population samples based on social variables predating, 68-78
  questionnaire design and, 66, 73
  ruling out physical and genetic explanations for, 75, 76
  search for causes of, 63-79
  social causes of, 66-71
  social policy and, 76-78
  social problems and mechanisms of, 67
  sociocultural disintegration, Stirling County Study, and, 186-189
  statistical analysis and, 74, 75
Psychiatric impairment
  adjustment and, 191-196
  anomia and,
    socioeconomic status, and, 198
    statistical analysis of, 199, 200
  epidemiology of, in normal populations, 186-189
  interrelations among anomia, social class and, 185-207
  major studies of, 186-204
  studies of social class and, 189-191
Psychiatric sociology
  cross-cultural research in
    data collection in, 86-89
    language barrier in, 85, 86

Psychiatric sociology—*continued*
    problems of, 81-103
    strategies and research models in, 83-86
disordered behavior, personality traits and, 31
framework for, 13-16
professional identity of, 9, 10
scope and theory of, 25-42
theoretical schemes and research problems in,
    29-35
Psychiatry
    adjoining service areas in community, 11-13
    sociology and, fusions and fissions of identity
        in, 5-17
Psychological autopsies, suicide and, 169

QUESTIONNAIRE design, psychiatric disorder
    and, 66, 73

REALITY, conception of, social class and, 129-
    131
Referral, psychiatric, labeling and/or, 46-50
Religion, suicide rates and, 168, 169
Research
    cross-cultural. *See* cross-cultural research.
    problems in, theoretical schemes and, 29-35
Role
    loss of, depression and, 146-155
    self-esteem and, 145
Role theory
    depression and, 144-146
    mental illness and sociopsychological, 44, 45

SCHIZOPHRENIA
    conceptions of reality and, 129
    definition and types of, 113, 114
    drift hypothesis and, 117-119
    direction of causality and, 117-121
    downward social mobility and, 118, 119
    ethnicity and, 122, 123
    genetics, stress and, 123-127
    hospital admissions and, 120
    indices for identity of, 120, 121
    isolation and, 34, 35, 123
    manic depression and, cultural variations in
        onset of, 35-39
    orientational systems and, 128, 130
    research model of, 131, 132
    social class and, 113-137
        family and, 127-129
        occupational mobility and, 116, 118, 119
        relationship of, 115, 116, 121-123
        social integration and, 122, 123
        stress relations and, 33
Second career stage, mental patient and, 46-50
Self-esteem
    impact of isolation on, 35
    role and, 145
Social causes of psychiatric disorder, 66-71

Social class
    conceptions of reality and, 129-131
    conformity and, 129-131
    definition of, 114
    depression and, 140, 141
    family, schizophrenia and, 127-129
    interrelations among anomia, psychiatric im-
        pairment and, 185-207
    measurement and comparability of social mo-
        bility and, 93-100
    mechanisms for relieving stress and, 126, 127
    orientational systems and, 129-131
    rates of hospital admission and, 120
    schizophrenia and, 113-137
        genetics and, 123-125
        relationship of, 115, 116, 121-123
        stress, and, 123, 125-127
        **studies of psychiatric impairment and, 189-
        191**
Social disruption, suicide and, 175, 176
Social gratification, mental disorder and de-
    ferment of, 191-195
Social integration, schizophrenia and, 122, 123
Social mobility
    measurement and comparability of social class
        and, 93-97
    schizophrenia and downward, 118, 119
Social policy, psychiatric disorder and, 76-78
Social problems, mechanisms of psychiatric
    disorder and, 67
Social psychiatry, definitional ambiguity of, 5-
    10
Social stability, Midtown Manhattan Study and
    analysis of, 30, 31
Social values, suicide and, 163
Social variables
    mechanisms for operation of, 76, 77
    predating psychiatric disorder, population
        samples based on, 68-78
Societies, classification of, in cross-cultural re-
    search, 89, 90
Sociocultural disintergration, psychiatric
    disorder, Stirling County Study, and, 186-
    189
Socioeconomic status
    Midtown Manhattan Study, anomia, and,
        186-189
    psychiatric impairment, anomia, and, 198
Sociological theories of suicide, 176-178
Sociology
    of depression, 139-157
    psychiatric. *See* Psychiatric sociology.
    psychiatry and, fusions and fissions on
        identity of, 5-17
    study of suicide and, 159-184
Statistics
    measuring anomia, psychiatric impairment
        and, 199, 200

212

Statistics—*continued*
    psychiatric disorder and, 74, 75
    misinterpretation of suicide, 170-173
    psychological autopsies and, 169
    suicide and, 164-178
Staff availability in cross-cultural research, 81-83
Stirling County Study, sociocultural disintergration, psychiatric disorder and, 186-187
Strategies, models and, in cross-cultural research, 83-86
Stress
    conceptions of reality and, 129-131
    schizophrenia and, 33, 123, 125-127
        genetics and, 124, 125
    social class and mechanisms for relieving, 126, 127
Suicide
    attemptors versus nonattemptors and, 181
    causes and dimensions of, 173-175
    classification of motives for, 166, 175
    cultural perception and, 179
    criticism and sociological study of, 162, 163
    Durkheim and, 160-164, 178, 179, 182
    ecological fallacy in study of, 163, 164
    psychological autopsies and, 169
    rates of
        coroners and, 173

    misinterpretation of, 170-173
    religion and, 168, 169, 172, 173
    social disruptions and, 175, 176
    social meanings of, 178-181
    sociological theories of, 176-178
    statistics and, 164-178
    stigma and, 167, 168
    study of, sociology and, 159-184
    understanding the victim and, 179-181
Surveys, critical interviews and instrument construction versus, 86-89
Sympathy, depression and, 146

THEORETICAL schemes and research problems in psychiatric sociology, 29-35
Theory-centered and problem-centered research, 31, 32
Third career stage, mental patient and, 51-58
Traditional roles of women, depression and, 140, 145, 154
Treatment, inpatient admission, discharge, and, 51-58

WOMEN
    depression and, 140, 142-152, 154, 155
    roles loss and, 140, 145, 147-155